T3-BHD-917

Occupational Therapy Evaluation

Obtaining and Interpreting Data

Jim Hinojosa, PHD, OT, FAOTA
Paula Kramer, PHD, OTR, FAOTA
—EDITORS—

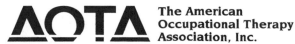

The American
Occupational Therapy
Association, Inc.

Occupational Therapy Evaluation: Obtaining and Interpreting Data is produced by the American Occupational Therapy Association. *Occupational Therapy Evaluation: Obtaining and Interpreting Data* may not be reproduced in whole or in part by any means without permission. For information, address The American Occupational Therapy Association, Inc., 4720 Montgomery Lane, PO Box 31220, Bethesda, MD 20824-1220.

The American Occupational Therapy Association, Inc. Mission Statement

The mission of the American Occupational Therapy Association is to support a professional community for members, and to develop and preserve the viability and relevance of the profession. The organization serves the interest of its members, represents the profession to the public, and promotes access to occupational therapy services.

Disclaimers

"This publication is designed to provide accurate and authoritative information in regard to the subject matter covered. It is sold or distributed with the understanding that the publisher is not engaged in rendering legal, accounting, or other professional services. If legal advice or other expert assistance is required, the services of a competent professional should be sought."

—*From the Declaration of Principles jointly adopted by the American Bar Association and a Committee of Publishers and Associations*

It is the objective of the American Occupational Therapy Association to be a forum for free expression and interchange of ideas. The opinions expressed by the contributors to this work are their own and not necessarily those of either the editors or the American Occupational Therapy Association.

AOTA Director of Nonperiodical Publications: Frances E. McCarrey
AOTA Managing Editor of Nonperiodical Publications: Mary C. Fisk
Text design by World Composition Services, Inc.
Cover design by Paul A. Platosh

ISBN 1-56900-090-5

Printed in the United States of America

This book is dedicated to
Raymond James Hinojosa
and
Rosalia A. Kramer
Though they are no longer with us,
their love, encouragement, and support continues in our hearts.

Contents

Contributors

Beatriz C. Abreu, PHD, OTR, FAOTA
Director of Occupational Therapy
Transitional Learning Community
    at Galveston
and
Clinical Professor
University of Texas Medical Branch
Galveston, Texas

Patricia Crist, PHD, OTR/L, FAOTA
Chair and Professor
Department of Occupational Therapy
Duquesne University
Pittsburgh, Pennsylvania

Cathy Dolhi, OTR/L
Associated Occupational Therapists, Inc.
Pittsburgh, Pennsylvania

Maureen Duncan, OTR/L
TheraPlayce Children's Developmental
    Center
Omaha, Nebraska
and
Doctoral Candidate, Occupational
    Therapy
Creighton University
School of Pharmacy & Allied Health
    Professions
Omaha, Nebraska

Winifred Dunn, PHD, OTR, FAOTA
Professor and Chair
Department of Occupational Therapy
    Education
School of Allied Health
University of Kansas Medical Center
Kansas City, Kansas

Rebecca Dutton, MS, OTR
Assistant Professor
Department of Occupational Therapy
Kean University
Union, New Jersey

Ruth Hansen, PHD, FAOTA
Department Head and Professor
Department of Associated Health
    Professions
Eastern Michigan University
Ypsilanti, Michigan

Jim Hinojosa, PHD, OT, FAOTA
Associate Professor
Department of Occupational Therapy
Director of Post-Professional Graduate
    Programs
New York University
New York, New York

**Cynthia Hughes Harris, PHD, OTR,
    FAOTA**
Columbia University
Programs in Occupational Therapy
New York, New York

Paula Kramer, PHD, OTR, FAOTA
Professor and Chair
Department of Occupational Therapy
Kean University
Union, New Jersey

**Mary Lou Leibold, MS,
    OTR/L**
Wexford, Pennsylvania

**Catherine Nielson, MPH, OT/L,
    FAOTA**
Clinical Associate Professor
Occupational Therapy Division
University of North Carolina at
    Chapel Hill
Chapel Hill, North Carolina

Jeannette Richards, OTR/L
Doctoral Candidate, Occupational
    Therapy
Creighton University

vii

School of Pharmacy & Allied Health
  Professions
Omaha, Nebraska

**Charlotte Brasic Royeen, PHD, OTR,
  FAOTA**
Professor and Associate Dean of Research
Creighton University
School of Pharmacy & Allied Health
  Professions
Omaha, Nebraska

Karen Stern, EDD, OTR
Associate Professor
Department of Occupational Therapy
Kean University
Union, New Jersey

Foreword

Changes in the evaluation process in occupational therapy reflect the evolution of the profession as a whole. In its early years, occupational therapy evaluation was relatively informal. Therapists gathered information from the physicians and the client, observed behavior, and selected a set of activities that would provide occupation that could be considered meaningful and restorative. Evaluation gradually became more structured, reflecting the theories and beliefs of each era. Thus in the 1950s and 1960s a number of projective assessments were designed, as a means to understand the unconscious conflicts of neurotic patients in psychiatric hospitals. As the 1960s passed, the first structured, standardized assessments of activities of daily living (ADL) appeared, focused primarily on inpatients in hospital settings, at that time the most typical site for care.

The 1960s and 1970s brought new emphasis on standardized, quantitative instruments that could provide "hard" data and could measure the progress of the individual. Some of these assessments were developed by occupational therapists, and some were borrowed from other professions. There was recognition that standardization was important, but most therapists admitted that they interpreted findings in ways consistent with personal beliefs and the perceived needs of the individual, rather than strictly by a set of rules.

The push for the development of standardized instruments became more intense in the 1980s as health care began the change still underway. Cost of care became an increasingly important factor, pressuring practitioners to measure carefully the starting point and progress for each individual. Without evidence of efficacy, the third–party payers (who most often covered the cost of care) were more and more likely to deny payment.

At the same time, several other important, interrelated trends have emerged. One is the belief that involvement of both the person and the family in the entire intervention process is highly desirable. Occupational therapists have espoused this view for some time, but have been reluctant to implement it formally in traditional health care settings where the physician has been in charge.

A second trend is the emphasis on quality of life. As the population has aged, it has become evident that perfect health is an unrealistic goal, so focus of care is shifting toward quality of life as the most desirable outcome. The Independent Living Movement demonstrated the interest of individuals with disabilities in ensuring that they would be able to undertake those activities of greatest value to them.

Third, care has moved rapidly away from inpatient settings. Outpatient treatment, partial hospitalization, and home health all have become increasingly important. At the same time length of inpatient stay is plummeting. Some of what had previously been considered health care moved out of the health care system entirely. For example, services for children with disabilities have shifted in large part to the school systems, where occupational therapists are now very frequently employed. Similarly, social service agencies developed options for patients discharged from psychiatric hospitals (at least insofar as any services were made available to such people).

These trends—accountability and cost containment, full engagement of the person in his or her treatment, emphasis on quality of life, and the movement away from inpatient care—have all contributed to significant changes in the ways that occupational therapists and other health care providers view the evaluation process.

Not surprisingly, evaluation has become much more complex. In some ways, it was easier to focus on standardized, quantitative assessments. It is, after all, more straightforward to measure range of motion than quality of life. However, most occupational therapists would acknowledge that the former is important only as it facilitates the latter.

Thus it is that we now find ourselves struggling to perfect an evaluation process that provides us with all the information that we and our clients require. The manifold pressures on our practice, coupled with our growing recognition of the needs of the individual, require us to employ an array of evaluation methods. We need to know about the activities that are meaningful to the individual, the environment in which those activities will occur, and the underlying performance components required for the person to accomplish those activities. We need to be able to determine what progress is being made. We need to know all this quickly and efficiently, because of all the costs involved. No small task.

We hope this book will be of value to therapists who find themselves struggling to provide the best possible care in a complicated world. While there are no simple choices or easy answers, it is essential that therapists know about the different means of evaluating their clients, as well as the many factors that affect choices made. It is essential that evaluation be based on a coherent theory that emphasizes the client's needs and wishes. Communication within the profession, with other professions, and with clients must be based on a common set of terms and understandings. Furthermore, evaluation must incorporate an array of assessment methods, both quantitative and qualitative, in order to be comprehensive and coherent. The competing interests of clients, payers, and care providers lead to legal and ethical issues that affect every decision made by the therapist.

There is another essential consideration. The current health care system is changing so rapidly, and has become so focused on costs and outcomes, that every profession in the system must justify its value in no uncertain terms. Years ago, it might have sufficed to have our clients express their gratitude and to "feel" that we had genuinely helped. Now, only hard data will suffice. This means research. Careful evaluation is at the core of research, whether in applied research examining outcomes of treatment, or in basic research examining the underlying premises and principles of occupation.

It is vital that therapists, researchers, and administrators have a single resource that can effectively address complex questions of evaluation, and we hope this book fills that role. This book also represents a source of considerable gratification for those of us who have watched the discipline grapple with the difficult issues over the years. Its various comprehensive contributions reflect the growing professional confidence that asserts our ability to evaluate not only our clients, but also the *means* by which we evaluate them. It is a great source of pleasure to read a volume that reflects so clearly the increasing maturity of a profession that is prepared to assert its own value and clarify its ability to develop its own practices and principles.

—Bette R. Bonder, PhD, OTR, FAOTA
Professor of Health Sciences and Psychology
Cleveland State University

Preface

At the February 1994 meeting of the Commission of Practice (COP) of the American Occupational Therapy Association (AOTA), the issue of assessment was discussed as there had been numerous calls from members to the National Office and the COP asking for clarification on the use of standardized tools, the evaluation process, and the documentation of findings. Furthermore, these members were concerned with the differentiation between the terms *assessment* and *evaluation*. Some occupational therapy educators also had asked for official guidance about when to use each term. The document entitled *Hierarchy of Competencies Relating to the Use of Standardized Instruments and Evaluation Techniques by Occupational Therapists* was rescinded by the Representative Assembly in 1992. While the *Hierarchy* document did define the terms *assessment* and *evaluation* from an AOTA perspective, it did not reflect current views of assessment in occupational therapy and did not reflect the growth in knowledge and information that is available about assessments.

Once the *Hierarchy* document was rescinded, the only remaining document that defined the terms of *assessment* and *evaluation* was the first edition of *Uniform Terminology for Reporting Occupational Therapy Services,* which was rescinded by the 1994 Representative Assembly. Subsequent editions of *Uniform Terminology* have not included a discussion of these terms; the Commission of Practice felt that the *Uniform Terminology* document is not the appropriate document in which to define these terms.

At its September 1994 meeting, COP members discussed how and when an occupational therapy practitioner should use the term *assessment* versus *evaluation*. Based on the first, rescinded edition of *Uniform Terminology,* occupational therapists were using *assessment* to refer to the entire process of determining the strengths and limitations of an individual client. The term *evaluation* was used when referring to specific tools or instruments that are used during the assessment process. COP noted that use of the terminology in this way was inconsistent with the way these terms were used in the physical therapy and speech–language pathology professions. Furthermore, a literature review revealed that the terms *evaluation* and *assessment* often are used interchangeably.

Based on these discussions and in order to facilitate consistency in all AOTA documents, the COP recommended that specific definitions be developed and that a text on evaluation be written. The COP then worked to develop an outline for such a text. This book is based on that outline. It is intended to clarify the distinct difference between evaluation and assessment as our profession has decided to use those terms. Furthermore, from a generic viewpoint, it presents the key issues about evaluation and assessment that all occupational therapy practitioners should know, from the theoretical basis of evaluation to documentation and further data use. It is our hope that this book will provide entry-level therapists with a comprehensive overview of evaluation and assessment.

Jim Hinojosa, PhD, OT, FAOTA
Paula Kramer, PhD, OTR, FAOTA

1 Evaluation— Where Do We Begin?

Jim Hinojosa, PHD, OT, FAOTA
Paula Kramer, PHD, OTR, FAOTA

Overview

This chapter outlines the unique reasons behind the creation of this book, focuses on defining evaluation and assessment, and serves as a guide to the rest of the book. Included in the chapter are a discussion of the role of the therapist in evaluation, the relationship between *Standards of Practice for Occupational Therapy* (AOTA, 1994a) (see Appendix A) and evaluation, and a discussion of ethics and professional judgment.

Introduction

A primary aspect of the occupational therapy process is evaluation. Findings or interpretation of evaluations determine the therapist's intervention strategies and course of actions. While occupational therapists have traditionally recognized the importance of evaluation, they have used the process and the terms associated with that process in an inconsistent manner. Distinctions generally have not been made among the terms associated with evaluation, assessment, specific tools, and the overall processes involved. Therapists have simply sought the information they want to obtain in order to determine whether there is

1

a need for intervention, rather than looking at what might be the optimal way of obtaining that information. They have not always looked at the whole process and how evaluation fits into the total scheme of practice. Occupational therapists need to give more attention to the evaluative process in a comprehensive way.

DEFINITIONS

Occupational therapists have frequently used the terms *evaluation* and *assessment* interchangeably. This can cause confusion since other professions have made distinctions between these terms. Therefore, in order to facilitate consistency in all American Occupational Therapy Association (AOTA) documents and with other professions, the Commission on Practice (COP) of AOTA recommended clarification of these terms. The delineation of these terms would be as follows:

> *Evaluation* refers to the overall process of obtaining and interpreting data necessary for understanding the individual, system, or situation. This includes planning for and documenting the process, results, and recommendations, including the need for intervention and/or potential change in the intervention plan.

> *Assessment* shall be used to refer to specific tools, instruments, or interactions that are used during the evaluation process. An assessment is a component part of the evaluation process.

While many professions continue to use these terms interchangeably, some have identified the distinction between evaluation and assessment in a different manner. The above definitions are meant to state the way these terms are used within the occupational therapy community. This is intended to help members of our profession communicate with each other more effectively, to increase our understanding of the evaluation and assessment processes, and to broaden our body of knowledge in this area.

THE FOCUS AND INTENT OF THIS TEXT

This book is intended to present and discuss the concepts of evaluation and assessment as they relate to individuals seeking occupational therapy services. It is not intended to review specific assessments or present evaluations with specific populations, though examples will be used. It will not deal with the complex topic of nonclient related evaluations in which occupational therapists engage, such as systems evaluations, facilities evaluations, or outcomes assessments. Instead, it will explore evaluation within the context of determining the need for intervention, and developing or changing the intervention plans.

As therapists, if we accept the premise that evaluations enable us to determine the need for intervention, and help us to develop a plan for intervention and understand when and how to change that plan, then we must fully understand this process in a manner that is broader than our understanding of the use of any specific assessment tool. The evaluative process is complex; it is fraught with clinical reasoning and decision making that will have a strong impact on interaction with consumers. This book is designed to facilitate a thorough understanding of this process.

The first section of this book will present general theoretical issues of evaluation. These include the theoretical basis of evaluation—its relationship to the philosophical basis of our profession and to frames of reference. The relationship between evaluation and the clinical reasoning process will be explored. Finally, this section will discuss how evaluation and assessment fits within the context of *Uniform Terminology for Occupational Therapy*, 3rd ed. (AOTA, 1994b) (see Appendix B).

The next section of this text will move into a more specific focus, exploring the evaluation process as it relates to both the client and the context. The various types of standardized and nonstandardized assessments used by occupational therapists will be reviewed, as well as how one goes about selecting appropriate assessment tools. The critical areas of evaluation interpretation, application, and documentation are presented.

Lastly, this book will examine legal and ethical issues of the evaluation process. Included in this section is a discussion on the overall use of evaluative data, particularly in research and outcomes analysis.

The Role of the Therapist in Evaluation

Professional education prepares practitioners for their therapeutic roles. According to the *Essentials and Guidelines for an Accredited Educational Program for the Occupational Therapist* (AOTA, 1991a), occupational therapy students are required to learn to select, administer, and interpret standardized and nonstandardized tests and assessments, in addition to making skilled observations, taking relevant histories, and interviewing clients and family members. Professional education prepares occupational therapists to evaluate individuals, to obtain and interpret data necessary for intervention, and to interpret evaluation findings to appropriate individuals (AOTA, 1993).

Many skills are needed to perform these tasks:

- a comprehensive knowledge of the domain of concern of the profession, human development and individual variation, and occupational roles and performance
- the ability to interact with the individual, to elicit information, and to be able to judge the client's performance and the quality of the response
- a broad repertoire of assessment tools and an understanding of the principles of tests and measurements

- a thorough understanding of the specific assessment tools selected, including strengths and limitations, psychometric properties, and applicability to specific situations
- the ability to put the data in the context of the individual's personal view of his or her life, environment, and chosen occupation.

The occupational therapy assistant (OTA) can participate in the evaluation process under the direction of the occupational therapist (AOTA, 1991b). At the entry level, the OTA assists with data collection and evaluation under the supervision of an OT (AOTA, 1993). At an intermediate level, the OTA administers standardized tests under the supervision of an OT after service competencies have been established (AOTA, 1993).

While the therapist must have this level of knowledge to be an evaluator, the therapist also must be able to put this knowledge into practice. The therapist should understand the circumstances of the evaluation that will influence the selection of the particular assessment tool. This includes the time allocated, space for evaluation, service delivery model, purpose of the evaluation, and the other evaluations being administered to the individual. Based on a knowledge of psychometrics as well as understanding of the individual, the therapist will make decisions about the use of reliable and valid assessments, the use of both subjective and objective data, understanding the differences between standardized and nonstandardized tools, as well as what will be most acceptable within the context of the evaluation. These factors will affect the choice of tools used in the evaluation. Simultaneously, the therapist should have the expertise and skills needed to administer the chosen assessments. Once the assessments have been administered, the therapist needs to interpret the data. This involves possibly combining data from several sources, determining what is important, and making clinical judgments about how these data fit with the domain of concern of occupational therapy. Following this, the therapist must document his or her findings in a format that is appropriate to the setting, and in a manner that is clear, concise, and understandable by all involved. In addition to documenting the evaluation, the therapist often must communicate the findings to the individual, to family or caregivers, or to other professionals. This should be done in a clear and accurate manner appropriate to the audience.

The process of evaluation is complex, involving many steps. At each step, the therapist must adhere to the *Standards of Practice for Occupational Therapy* (AOTA, 1994a). Following *Standards of Practice,* the first step is screening. Screening provides a preliminary overview of the individual, his or her needs, assets and limitations, and whether or not a more complete evaluation is necessary. Based on these data, the therapist can do an analysis of potential problems, which can be explored through a comprehensive evaluation. It is the responsibility of the therapist to choose appropriate tools for the evaluation.

This requires the therapist to have vast knowledge of the various assessments available, to know which are appropriate, and to be flexible in choosing assessment tools, rather than relying on a few favorite instruments.

During evaluation, therapists must continuously review the data as they come in and then make appropriate decisions and judgments. This process has been described as "intensive" and "dynamic," requiring constant rethinking and decision-making as each assessment is presented and then completed (Kramer, 1993). Once each task or activity is completed, the therapist must decide how to proceed. Each decision then leads to another set of choices (such as using another assessment), until the therapist has gathered enough information to draw conclusions. This type of decision tree is very similar to the deductive analysis approach used in clinical research in nursing; however, it also can be seen as a process of analysis and reordering of diagnostic elements in an evaluative conclusion (Jones, 1988). It is an excellent example of the "thinking in action process" described by Schon (1983), who studied how numerous health professionals continually reflect on their performance and decisions while they practice.

A therapist's clinical reasoning is influenced by the way he or she views the overall evaluation process, which is itself based on the way we view practice. Occupational therapists do not have one accepted way of conceptualizing practice; there are many schools of thought. Some scholars advocate particular models; some offer distinct paradigms; and others focus on frames of reference. In this book, frames of reference are used frequently as a way of conceptualizing practice. Regardless of how practice is conceptualized, though, evaluation is always an integral part of the model, the paradigm, or the frame of reference. This text is intended to explore evaluation in depth, so that one can then apply this knowledge within his or her own practice.

While these differing perspective exist, the profession has clearly defined and accepted its scope of practice. *Uniform Terminology for Occupational Therapy,* 3rd ed. (AOTA, 1994b) provides a generic outline and identifies the domain of concern of the profession:

> *Performance areas* are broad categories of human activity that are typically part of daily life. They are activities of daily living, work and productive activities, and play or leisure activities.

> *Performance components* are fundamental human abilities that—to varying degrees and in differing combinations—are required for successful engagement in performance areas. These components are sensorimotor, cognitive, psychosocial and psychological.

> *Performance contexts* are situations or factors that influence an individual's engagement in desired and/or required performance areas.

Performance contexts consist of *temporal* aspects (chronological age, developmental age, place in life cycle, and health status), and *environmental* aspects (physical, social, and cultural considerations) (pp. 1–2).

It is recognized that performance components and performance contexts interact and may have an impact on performance areas. Both performance components and performance contexts are looked at based on how they influence the individual's abilities to function within performance areas. For a complete delineation of performance areas, performance components, and performance contexts, see Appendix B, *Uniform Terminology for Occupational Therapy,* 3rd ed. (AOTA, 1994b).

Whatever the therapist's conceptualization of practice, there are generally three ways of approaching evaluation based on *Uniform Terminology* (1994b). One way focuses first on the performance areas, another focuses first on the performance components, and another focuses first on the performance context.

EVALUATIONS THAT BEGIN WITH THE PERFORMANCE AREAS

When the focus is on the performance area, the therapist usually looks broadly at activities of daily living, work and productive activities, and play or leisure activities. Functional assessments are used to determine the individual's abilities and problem areas. In this approach, the client directs the evaluation by identifying occupations and activities that are important, and the therapist looks at the client's abilities relative to those occupations. The next step involves looking at underlying performance components that may be deficient and in need of intervention to allow the individual to successfully engage in meaningful activities. The therapist then considers the performance context. The resultant documentation of the evaluation includes the description of those activities that the individual is able to perform, those that are difficult for the individual, the underlying deficient performance components, and an identification of where intervention may be needed.

Case Example

Joe is a 48-year-old male who is 1 week post CVA and is medically stable. He was referred to occupational therapy for a complete evaluation and intervention. The therapist reads the medical documentation as part of a screening process and meets the patient. Given the therapist's initial data gathering and Joe's concerns, the therapist focuses first on activities of daily living. Her evaluation explores Joe's ability to feed, bathe, toilet, and dress himself. Through functional activities and specific assessments, such as the Functional Independence Measure (FIM) (Hamilton, Granger, Sherwin, et al., 1987), the therapist determines his ability to engage in this performance area. Once the therapist determines that Joe has a problem with this performance area, she then may evaluate specific performance components, such as manual muscle testing and range of motion, to gain more information about how these performance components might be affecting this performance area. Then, with consideration to the performance context, a plan for intervention can be developed. ■

EVALUATIONS THAT START WITH PERFORMANCE COMPONENTS

An alternative way of approaching evaluation is to begin by evaluating specific performance components. When the focus is on the performance components, the therapist looks specifically at basic foundational elements such as sensorimotor, cognitive, or psychosocial. This may be done through specific assessments or tools that pinpoint these particular concerns. The therapist, in this approach, directs the evaluation towards a focus on specific performance components. Then the therapist looks at the results of these assessments and determines the relationship of deficient performance components to the more general performance areas and the performance context. The resultant documentation of the evaluation includes the performance components that may need intervention, how those specific performance components relate to and affect ability to engage in activities representative of the performance areas in context, and where intervention may be needed.

Case Example

Mariko, a 4-year-old child, was referred to occupational therapy because of suspected developmental delay. After reading the referral documentation and getting an overview of the child through a discussion with the child's care providers, the occupational therapist decides to assess her gross and fine motor skills, muscle tone, movement patterns, manipulation skills, and give a standardized assessment, the Miller Assessment for Preschoolers (MAP) (Miller, 1982). Once the therapist identifies those performance components that are interfering with Mariko's functional abilities through clinical observation and the data obtained from the MAP, he or she then ascertains which performance areas are affected. Following this, and considering the performance context, a plan for intervention can be developed. ■

The purpose in beginning the evaluation with the performance components is to determine what personal variables might be contributing to or creating barriers to desired performance. Therefore, the therapist combines the data gained from the clinical observations of Mariko's gross and fine motor skills, muscle tone, movement patterns, and manipulation skills, with the data gained from the MAP. Once the therapist identifies those performance components that are interfering with Mariko's functional abilities through clinical observation and the data obtain from the MAP, he or she ascertains which performance areas are affected. The therapist then focuses on assessing her functional skills, abilities, and experiences. For this aspect of evaluation, the occupational therapist assesses abilities in the performance areas relative to the performance context.

EVALUATIONS THAT START WITH PERFORMANCE CONTEXT

Another way of approaching evaluation is to begin by evaluating the performance context. When the focus is on the performance context, the therapist evaluates the person relative to the disability status, lifestyle, age, and stage of life, as well as setting and environment. The therapist considers possible supports and barriers to performance, based upon context, and assesses performance components and the performance areas. The resultant documentation of the evaluation includes extensive consideration of the differences in performance based upon context. Therapeutic interventions are based on typical performance needs.

Case Example

Muhammad is a 72-year-old male recovering from an aneurysm that resulted in mild motor deficits. He was referred to occupational therapy for an ADL evaluation prior to being admitted to a skilled nursing facility. After reading the referral documentation, the occupational therapist decides to assess Muhammad's performance of daily life activities, considering what he wants and what he will need to do at the skilled nursing facility. The therapist interviews Muhammad and observes the skilled nursing facility. She finds out that before his hospitalization, Muhammad had lived alone and that he is now fearful of returning to his apartment. Given his age and his lifestyle, along with his newly acquired disability, he feels that he would be comfortable in a skilled nursing facility that has some assisted living residences within it. This will allow him to move into those residences if his condition improves. He has chosen this particular setting because it is respectful of his cultural background, and he believes that he will feel comfortable with the people there. The data from the assessment of the performance context provide the background upon which the therapist assesses the performance areas and the performance components. Based upon all the data, an intervention plan is developed for Muhammad that focuses on developing his ability to function within the skilled nursing facility, with the potential of having him eventually move to a less restrictive environment. ■

STARTING THE EVALUATION

While therapists may have the choice of which way to approach an evaluation, at times the type or focus of the evaluation may be determined externally. The institution may require that a specific assessment be used or that an evaluation include specific assessments. For example, a hospital may require that all clients on the inpatient unit be evaluated using the *Bay Area Functional Performance Evaluation, 2nd ed.* (Williams & Bloomer, 1987). A service delivery model may require a specific focus on the evaluation, such as a school system, which requires that evaluations focus on educational relevancy. In other circumstances, a referral may suggest or require a specific type of evaluation, such as a referral for occupational therapy following joint replacement surgery. Regardless of whether the therapist has a choice in the evaluation process or the tools used, the therapist has a professional responsibility to ensure that the overall evaluation meets the needs of the consumer and reflects the domain of concern of occupational therapy.

Another important influence on the type and focus of evaluation is the consumer. It is incumbent on the therapist to listen to the consumer and respond appropriately. At times this requires teaching the consumer about his or her condition and the role of occupational therapy. The consumer may have specific concerns or expectations, such as the individual who wants to be independent in bathing and toileting but does not care if he or she needs help with dressing. In this case the therapist has two options: to only evaluate and address the performance areas that are of concern to the client, or to educate the client about areas that may be improved or enhanced through therapy. It should be noted that the consumer has the right to refuse evaluation or intervention.

The informed consumer can bring his or her own concerns, ideas, and expectations of what will be included in the evaluation process and what outcomes are expected. The therapist may or may not agree with the consumer's perspective. However, it is critical that the therapist involve the consumer and consider his or her point of view. Open discussion about the evaluation and the concerns of both parties will serve as the basis for a positive therapeutic relationship. Through this collaboration, the therapist and the consumer can reach a consensus on the evaluation, its focus, and its scope. An open, trusting relationship established during the evaluation can serve as the foundation for future intervention.

In summary, the role of the occupational therapist in evaluation is complex, requiring both knowledge and skills. Basic academic education provides a core understanding. However, throughout one's professional career, this understanding will be expanded through proficiency, mastery, and continued learning.

STANDARDS OF PRACTICE

AOTA has adopted *Standards of Practice* (1994a), which are recommended guidelines for the provision of occupational therapy service. These are considered the *minimum* standard for practice; therefore, advanced practice may go beyond these standards. Two specific standards relate to the broad area of evaluation: Standard III, screening; and Standard IV, assessment (to be revised to evaluation). Therapists should be aware of the *Standards of Practice* in their entirety and should not take those related to evaluation out of context of the whole document, even though only two of the standards are presented here.

Standard III: Screening

The process of evaluation begins with screening: a preliminary overview of the individual to determine the need for a complete evaluation or to make other recommendations, such as the need for involvement of another professional.

1. A registered occupational therapist, in accordance with state and federal guidelines, shall conduct screening to determine whether intervention or further assessment is necessary and to identify dysfunctions in occupational performance areas.
2. A registered occupational therapist shall screen independently or as a member of an interdisciplinary team. A certified occupational therapy assistant may contribute to the screening process under the supervision of a registered occupational therapist.
3. A registered occupational therapist shall select screening methods that are appropriate to the individual's age and developmental level; gender; education; cultural background; and socioeconomic, medical, and functional status. Screening methods may include, but are not limited to, interviews, structured observations, informal testing, and record reviews.
4. A registered occupational therapist shall communicate screening results and recommendations to appropriate individuals.

(AOTA, 1994A, 1039–1040)

Standard IV: Assessment (evaluation)

Evaluation is the process of obtaining and interpreting data necessary for understanding the individual. This includes the entire process, from gathering data through interpreting them, documenting findings, and communicating results to the individual and to appropriate persons.

1. A registered occupational therapist shall assess an individual's occupational performance components and occupational performance areas. A registered occupational therapist conducts assessments individually or as part of a team of professionals, as appropriate to the practice settings and the purposes of the assessments. A certified occupational therapy assistant may contribute to the assessment process under the supervision of a registered occupational therapist.

2. An occupational therapy practitioner shall educate the individual, or the individual's family or legal guardian, as appropriate, about the purposes and procedures of the occupational therapy assessment.

3. A registered occupational therapist shall select assessments to determine the individual's functional abilities and problems as related to occupational performance areas' occupational performance components, physical, social, and cultural environments; performance safety; and prevention of dysfunction.

4. Occupational therapy assessment methods shall be appropriate to the individual's age and developmental level; gender; education; socioeconomic, cultural, and ethnic background; medical status; and functional abilities. The assessment methods may include some combination of skilled observation, interview, record review, or the use of standardized or criterion-referenced tests. A certified occupational therapy assistant may contribute to the assessment process under the supervision of a registered occupational therapist.

5. An occupational therapy practitioner shall follow accepted protocols when standardized tests are used. Standardized tests are tests whose scores are based on accompanying normative data that may reflect age ranges, gender, ethnic groups, geographic regions, and socioeconomic status. If standardized tests are not available or appropriate, the results shall be expressed in descriptive reports, and standardized scales shall not be used.

6. A registered occupational therapist shall analyze and summarize collected evaluation data to indicate the individual's current functional status.

7. A registered occupational therapist shall document assessment results in the individual's records, noting the specific evaluation methods and tools used.

8. A registered occupational therapist shall complete and document results of occupational therapy assessments within the time frames established by practice settings, government agencies, accreditation programs, and third-party payers.

9. An occupational therapy practitioner shall communicate assessment results, within the boundaries of client confidentiality, to the appropriate persons.

10. A registered occupational therapist shall refer the individual to the appropriate services or request additional consultation if the results of the assessments indicate areas that require intervention by other professionals.

(AOTA, 1994a, 1040)

Ethics and Professional Judgment

Principle Three of the *Occupational Therapy Code of Ethics* (AOTA, 1994c) (see Appendix C) states that "Occupational therapy personnel shall achieve and continually maintain high standards of competence" (p. 1037). An entry-level occupational therapist cannot be expected to be competent in all the assessments that occupational therapists use; however, it is imperative that the therapist be competent in the administration and interpretation of an assessment before using it with a client. To achieve this competency, the therapist should read about the evaluation, understand its unique purpose, understand the psychometric properties involved, know whether it requires the use of standardized procedures, and have adequate knowledge and skills to perform these procedures. When considering the use of an unfamiliar assessment tool, it is recommended that the therapist discuss the tool with others who are more knowledgeable in its use, in order to learn more about its assets and limitations. Standardized assessments require that the therapist be rigorous in following administration procedures. It is important to rehearse the administration of the assessment and to learn what are acceptable variations of performance. As always, it is the therapist's professional responsibility to make sure that he or she is competent in the use of a tool before using it with a client.

Some assessment tools are not designed for usage by the entry-level occupational therapist. These tools require certification, postprofessional continuing education, and/or additional academic degrees. Some examples are the *Sensory Integration and Praxis Tests* (SIPT) (Ayres, 1989), *Assessment of Motor and Process Skills* (AMPS) (Fischer, 1992), *Bailey Scales of Infant Development, 2nd ed.* (Bailey, 1994), and *Wechsler Preschool and Primary Scale of Intelligence* (Wechsler, 1967). Therapists often choose to seek out postprofessional education that will develop the skills and competencies necessary to use specialized assessment tools. It is a professional responsibility that the therapist make certain that he or she has the necessary skills and underlying knowledge before using specialized tools. Further, it is essential that the therapist accurately represent his or her background in these assessments to clients. When therapists select specialized tests that are more frequently associated with other disciplines, they have the additional challenge and responsibility to make sure that their interpretation of these instruments reflects the domain of concern of occupational therapy.

Both standardized and nonstandardized assessment tools are designed for specific situations, such as for specific populations or age groups, for those individuals who share a particular background, or for people who are fluent in one language. When a tool is used with another population, or with people from a different culture, the results may not necessarily be the same, or even valid. In such a situation, areas identified as deficits may not actually be deficits.

All tests have biases. It is critical for therapists to recognize the biases in the assessment tools that they use. Biases can occur in gender, educational level, socio-economic background, ethnic background, cultural background, geographic environment, or medical status. Because the occupational therapist is concerned with the person's everyday life and the performance of daily tasks, the occupational therapist should gather information about the individual and his or her background and culture, in order to select an appropriate tool that will suit that particular individual, rather than just meet the needs of an average person of the same age or diagnosis. For example, if the therapist receives a referral to evaluate a person with right hemiplegia, the therapist first needs to investigate the person's age, gender, culture, interests, goals, and other factors that influence him or her, in order to gain a better understanding of the types of occupations in which this person engages. Based upon such information, the therapist can choose an appropriate assessment tool.

No single assessment tool should be the basis for determining a problem area. The use of multiple tools helps the therapist to avoid test bias, as well as gives a better picture of the variations that may occur in an individual's performance. Therapists frequently find that the use of a combination of standardized and nonstandardized instruments, combined with observations and clinical judgment, provide an overall portrait of the individual's strengths and limitations. Additionally, when the therapist shares his or her hypotheses with the team, an enhanced view of the client may result. Each member of the team contributes a different perspective, and, through the information gained from the collaborative process of the team, a complete picture of the person's abilities and disabilities can emerge.

The *Occupational Therapy Code of Ethics* (1994c) states that occupational therapy practitioners shall protect the confidential nature of information obtained from an individual. All information gained during the evaluation process should be considered confidential. When multiple professionals are evaluating an individual, it is also very helpful for professionals to keep their findings and interpretations confidential from each other until all personnel have completed their evaluations. This infra-team confidentiality can prevent one person from being unduly swayed by the hypotheses of another, ensuring a more objective conclusion. It can also help the team to identify variations in the individual's performance from one evaluation session to another.

In most cases, the evaluation process is not complete until the findings have been written into an evaluation report or evaluation summary. These reports should be concise, yet comprehensive. Therapists should be careful not to over-interpret data or suggest results that may still be inconclusive. It is also important that occupational therapy evaluation summaries should reflect the domain of concern of occupational therapy and identify strengths and limitations related to the occupational performance areas of the individual. The point of the report is to communicate information. The therapist needs to know the audience when constructing the report. The consumer may need a report that is written with an educational focus, while a physician may need the data in a succinct, professional manner; and a third-party payer may require an altogether different set of information. This may necessitate more than one summary being written on the same client. In any case, it is often prudent to avoid jargon and complex language. Reports should be proofread to ensure correct spelling and grammar and to eliminate awkward sentences that would be unclear to the reader. Finally, formal reports, and particularly those going outside of the institution, should be formatted and typed in a professional style. The professional presentation of a report often determines the first impression.

Summary

A primary aspect of the occupational therapy process is evaluation. Client-based evaluation in occupational therapy is conceptualized around the profession's domain of concern: performance components, performance areas, and performance context. Accepting that there are many ways of conceptualizing practice, occupational therapists generally approach evaluating clients by starting assessment of any aspect of the profession's domain of concern. However, comprehensive evaluation requires that occupational therapists assess all aspects of the domain of concern as they relate to the individual client. In the occupational therapist's role as an evaluator, he or she must comply with the AOTA's *Standards of Practice* (1994a), the *Code of Ethics* (1994c), and sound professional judgment.

References

American Occupational Therapy Association. (1991a). Essentials and guidelines for an accredited educational program for the occupational therapist. *American Journal of Occupational Therapy, 45,* 1077–1084.

American Occupational Therapy Association. (1991b). Essentials and guidelines for an accredited educational program for the occupational therapy assistants. *American Journal of Occupational Therapy, 45.* 1085–1092.

American Occupational Therapy Association. (1993). Occupational therapy roles. *American Journal of Occupational Therapy, 47.* 1087–1105.

American Occupational Therapy Association. (1994a). Standards of practice for occupational therapy. *American Journal of Occupational Therapy, 48.* 1039–1043.

American Occupational Therapy Association. (1994b). Uniform terminology for occupational therapy (3rd ed.). *American Journal of Occupational Therapy, 48.* 1047–1054.

American Occupational Therapy Association. (1994c). Occupational therapy code of ethics. *American Journal of Occupational Therapy, 48.* 1037–1038.

Ayres, A.J. (1989). *Sensory integration and praxis tests.* Los Angeles: Western Psychological Services.

Bailey, N. (1994). *Bailey scales of infant development* (2nd. ed.). San Antonio, TX: Psychological Corporation.

Fisher, A.G. (1992). *Assessment of motor and process skills* (Res. ed. 6.1J). Unpublished test manual, Department of Occupational Therapy, Fort Collins, CO: Colorado State University.

Jones, J. (1988). Clinical reasoning in nursing. *Journal of Advanced Nursing. 13,* 185–192.

Kramer, P. (1993). *Pediatric occupational therapists' views of their procedures and practices when evaluating children.* Unpublished doctoral dissertation, New York University, NY.

Miller, L.J. (1982). *The Miller assessment for preschoolers.* Littleton, CO: Foundation for Knowledge in Development.

Schon, D. (1983). *The reflective practitioner: How professionals think in action.* New York, NY: Basic Books.

Wechsler, D. (1967). *Wechsler preschool and primary scale of intelligence.* San Antonio, TX: Psychological Corporation.

Williams, S.L., & Bloomer, J. (1987). *Bay Area functional performance evaluation administration and scoring manual* (2nd. ed.). Palo Alto, CA: Consulting Psychologist.

2 Theoretical Basis of Evaluation

Paula Kramer, PHD, OTR, FAOTA
Jim Hinojosa, PHD, OT, FAOTA

Overview

As an important component of the occupational therapy process, evaluation is based on the philosophical assumptions and beliefs of the profession. This chapter presents the philosophical basis of evaluation, as well as the theoretical basis of evaluation and assessments. It continues with the relationship among theory, evaluation, and practice, and a discussion of clinical reasoning in evaluation.

Introduction: Philosophical Foundation of Evaluation

All professions have philosophical beliefs that guide what that profession feels is important. These beliefs have an impact on what the professional does and on how he or she evaluates and determines the focus of the intervention. These beliefs form the unique philosophical foundation of a profession, an underlying set of premises or principles that may be facts, beliefs, values, or assumptions. The philosophical foundation of occupational therapy guides therapists in their actions, including the selection of evaluation tools or assessments. Furthermore, our philosophical foundation influences how assessments

17

are used. Some of the basic philosophical beliefs of our profession focus on how we view the individual and his or her rights. Occupational therapists believe that an individual:

- has the right to a meaningful existence
- is influenced by the biological and social nature of the species
- can only be understood within the context of family, friends, community, and cultural group membership
- has the need to participate in a variety of social roles and to have periodic relief from participation
- has the right to seek his or her potential through personal choice within the context of accepted social constraints
- is able to reach his or her potential through purposeful interaction with the human and nonhuman environment (Mosey, 1996).

Additionally, occupational therapists have strong beliefs about the importance of occupations and activities; therefore, they believe that individuals have an occupational nature and that occupation is necessary to society and culture. Occupational therapists believe that occupation is required for physical and psychological well-being, and personal occupations are a product of one's development (Keilhofner, 1992). All of these beliefs influence the way occupational therapists look at individuals, the way in which they will evaluate those individuals, and the areas in which the occupational therapists will intervene. Thus, an occupational therapy evaluation always considers:

- the individual's biological and personal development
- the individual's cultural and social context
- the individual's relationship with family and significant others
- the individual's engagement in personal occupations
- the quality of the individual's performance in personal occupation
- the individual's personal occupations in relationship to the physical and psychological development.

In addition to the basic philosophical beliefs that influence how occupational therapists look at individuals, occupational therapists also have some basic beliefs about evaluation in general. Four of these beliefs are:

1. Evaluation is an ongoing process that starts when the individual is first referred to the therapist and continues throughout intervention to discharge (Stewart, 1996).
2. Assessments have potential biases that may influence their usefulness and appropriateness with selected groups of individuals.
3. An assessment of an individual includes his or her perspective as well as those of the family, significant others, and/or caregivers.

4. The documented evaluation should include a comprehensive picture of the individual's occupational roles, performances areas, performance components, and functional skills and abilities.

Evaluation is an ongoing process that starts when the individual is first referred to the therapist and continues throughout intervention to discharge (Stewart, 1996). Though evaluation is sometimes discussed as a discrete segment, it is actually part of the continuum of intervention. It is an interactive process with a client that is dynamic in nature. Both therapist and client shape the evaluation through their input, interaction, and responses to each other, as well as to the assessments or activities that are presented. While the therapist starts with a formalized evaluation, evaluation continues throughout the intervention process. The therapist will continually monitor the person's response to intervention and gather data about any changes. This ongoing evaluation may be less formalized. This overview of evaluation highlights that evaluation begins with the first contact with the individual and continues until the individual is discharged from therapy.

Therapists spend great effort evaluating their clients through intervention and are concerned with obtaining reliable and valid data. The formal evaluation provides a baseline of the individual's performance. From this baseline, with ongoing evaluation, the therapist determines the client's specific needs for intervention and can continually observe whether progress is being made and whether a change in programming is needed.

Assessments have potential biases that may influence their usefulness and appropriateness with selected groups of individuals. Occupational therapists are aware that all assessments may have some degree of bias. The most obvious biases are related to culture, gender, geographic area, and socioeconomic status. With standardized assessments, the bias may come from the use of a homogeneous population when the tool was standardized. It may also come from items that are specific to one cultural group or gender or to a region of the country.

Another type of bias is personal or examiner bias that may be conscious or unconscious (King-Thomas, 1987). One type of examiner bias is based on expectations: If the evaluation is performed on someone who is poorly dressed and wearing soiled clothes, the examiner may not expect that person to do well on the evaluation. Though we may have difficulty acknowledging them, all people, including therapists, have some prejudices. Personal prejudices should be explored, so that they do not interfere with professional judgments. Additionally, therapists sometimes have preconceived notions based on their background or prior experiences. When one reads a diagnosis in a chart, one may expect certain characteristics, which may or may not be present. The therapist needs to be aware of what is actually being observed, rather than what he or she might expect to observe. While reading a chart and becoming familiar with the client's history is part of good practice, the therapist needs to be able to keep that information separate from data-gathering and conclusions.

An assessment of an individual includes his or her perspective as well as those of the family, significant others, and caregivers. An individual cannot be evaluated in isolation. For an occupational therapist to understand the individual, he or she must collect data from the individual's significant others. This will give the therapist another, useful perspective on the individual, and his or her ability to engage in meaningful activities. Occupational therapy is concerned with the functional performance of the individual in daily life. This includes not only what the person can or cannot do, but also how he or she functions in the environment, including involvement with others.

The documented evaluation should include a comprehensive picture of the individual's occupational roles, performances areas, performance components, and functional skills and abilities. Written evaluations need to be complete, providing others with important information about the total person's life and lifestyle, and those occupations and activities that are important to him or her. It should not be limited to discussing one performance component or performance area. Occupational therapy evaluation narratives should reflect the values of the profession, while providing an integrated portrait of the person's life. The evaluations ongoing through the intervention process should state the focus of intervention and highlight the functional changes that occur as intervention progresses.

In summary, our philosophy defines who we are and what our focus is; it guides our practice, identifying what is important to us, what we will assess, and how we will intervene. It makes our contribution to society unique.

Theoretical Basis of Assessments

Based on the understanding of the impact of the philosophical beliefs on the evaluation process, it is critical to explore the impact of theory on evaluation. Our philosophical beliefs will guide, to some extent, those theories that are applicable to or appropriate for the profession to use. The theories that occupational therapists choose to use must be consistent with the philosophy of the profession.

Theories are a collection of concepts, definitions, and postulates that are organized so as to make predictions about the relationship among events. Concepts are labels describing observed phenomena. The meaning of important concepts are their definitions. The stated relationships between two or more concepts are postulates (Kramer & Hinojosa, 1993). It is incumbent upon the person who develops a theory to identify and define the concepts and state the postulates. In this way, the theorist determines the scope and parameters of the theory. A theory organizes information in a way that is understandable, explaining the relationships between ideas and observed events in a logical manner. It links all the various concepts, definitions, and principles in a coherent way. Theories are critical to the foundation of any type of intervention, and, therefore, theories are basic to evaluation. Theory plays a role in the conceptualization of most assessment tools.

Most assessment tools explore performance relative to the areas of concern of a particular theory. When occupational therapists choose an assessment, they need to be aware of the theory or theories according to which that tool is designed. Theories define the concepts and relationships that are selected to develop the instrument and determine what will be included in the instrument. They also establish the parameters for the appropriate use of the instrument, including what is important to assess and how it will be assessed. For example, a developmental theory is concerned with stage-specific milestones in gross and fine motor areas. Following this theory, developmental milestones are defined as acceptable parameters for achieving certain gross and fine motor tasks. An instrument based on this theory might be a checklist of tasks and the acceptable parameters for the achievement of each task. Almost all instruments have some conceptual rationale for how the test is constructed, what is included within it, and how it should be used.

Ideally, there would be a wide variety of assessment tools, based on the theories and philosophies that are important to occupational therapy. This would allow occupational therapists to choose assessments for an evaluation based on the theory most applicable to the individual. It would also ensure that the tool would fit with our concern with performance areas, performance components, and performance context. We should be aware that while some assessments are based on theories that fit neatly with the philosophical beliefs of occupational therapy, there are many more that were developed from other theoretical orientations even though they may relate to our concerns. Occupational therapists always have the challenge of selecting and interpreting the information obtained from an assessment tools so that it is consistent with their own professional concerns and beliefs. For example, the *Bruininks-Oseretsky Test of Motor Proficiency* (Bruininks, 1978) was developed for use in special education. However, occupational therapists use this tool, because it gives a good picture of gross and fine motor skills, as well as bilateral integration and balance, especially with older children. Occupational therapists feel comfortable using this test because it is consistent with their philosophy.

Other factors influence which particular assessment tools are to be used. Some are used because they are popular. Others are used because they are valued by other professions. Some are used because they are standardized, and such data are required by certain settings. Some are used because they are required by an institution, regulations, or particular service delivery model. Under these circumstances, the occupational therapist has the responsibility to translate the information into the domain of concern of the profession.

The application of theory to practice is a complex process. The therapist is obliged to take abstract ideas and apply them. As previously stated, there are several acceptable ways of conceptualizing occupational therapy practice. In each of these, evaluation is an important component and serves as the basis for intervention. Some of the more common ones are:

- frames of reference (Bruce & Borg, 1993, 1987; Kramer & Hinojosa, 1993; Mosey, 1970, 1981, 1986, 1992, 1996)
- models (Reed & Sanderson, 1992)
- conceptual models of practice (Keilhofner, 1992)
- conceptual systems for guiding practice (Christiansen, 1991) and
- guidelines for practice (Mosey, 1996).

All of these vehicles allow practitioners to utilize theory as the basis for their evaluations and interventions. In this book, we will use frames of reference as the way of conceptualizing practice, to illustrate the evaluative process.

Theory, Evaluation, and Practice

Evaluation and intervention should always be based on the use of theory. Theory and practice need to be continually linked. There are four major considerations involved in relating theory to evaluation and practice:

1. the individual
2. screening and determining the appropriate frame(s) of reference
3. choosing the frame of reference and assessment(s)
4. intervention/treatment planning and implementation

The importance of the individual in the evaluation process is discussed throughout this book. The evaluation begins with the individual, considering his or her life experiences, life roles, interests and occupations, age, cultural background, and situational context.

The process of determining whether an individual needs intervention, and then, which frame of reference is most appropriate, involves three major steps. The first is to screen the individual so that one can make an educated decision as to the person's potential need for service. The second step involves determining whether the individual's needs fit within the domain of occupational therapy. The third step is to decide which frame(s) of reference would be most suitable for the individual's needs. Each step offers choices for the therapist to make and requires clinical reasoning.

The initial screening process involves looking at the individual's needs, strengths, limitations, and environment. The purpose of initial screening is to obtain an overview of the individual; it is not meant to be a comprehensive evaluation. Screenings may involve an observation of the individual, a chart review, medical and developmental history, the information gained from parents or care providers, or data gathered by other professionals (Collier, 1991). Additionally, the therapist may administer standardized or nonstandardized screening tools such as the Denver II Developmental Screening Test (Frankenberg, Dodds, Archer, Bresnick, Maschka, Edelman, & Shapiro, 1991), Clinical Observations of Neuromuscular Integration (Ayres, 1976), Family Observation Guide (Hinojosa & Kramer, 1996), Activity Configuration (Mosey, 1986), Interest Checklist (Matsutsuyu, 1969), Occupational History (Moorehead, 1969), Autonomic Nervous System Inventory (Farber, 1982), and Functional Status Questionnaire (Jette, Davis, Cleary, et al., 1986). By gathering useful information through the screening process, the therapist is able to determine what approach or frame of reference will best meet the individual's and family's needs, rather than choosing one that is purely based on the therapist's preference.

From the screening, the therapist has a preliminary picture and begins to understand what occupational therapy might offer this person. The second step of this process involves exploring the needs of the individual as they relate to the domain of concern of occupational therapy. This helps the therapist decide whether or not occupational therapy is appropriate for this particular individual. If the therapist determines that another service is needed, a referral should be made. If the therapist decides that occupational therapy is not necessary, the individual should be discharged.

The screening data can now be viewed with an understanding of what occupational therapy can offer this individual. The primary concern of occupational therapists is that an individual be able to function in the performance areas. It is recognized that performance components and performance contexts interact and may have an impact on performance areas. Both performance components and performance contexts are based on how they influence the individual's abilities to function within performance areas. For a complete delineation of performance areas, performance components, and performance contexts, see Appendix B, *Uniform Terminology for Occupational Therapy,* 3rd ed. (AOTA, 1994).

At this point, the therapist is ready to choose the most appropriate frame of reference for the individual. Several factors should be taken into consideration. The first and most important are the needs of the individual and the outcomes desired by that person and his or her family. For example, an individual who needs to learn to dress himself may be best served by a therapist using a frame of reference that is based on learning theories. Another example is the child who is just learning to make the transition from one position to another. His parents' goal is for him to be able to crawl. The therapist might choose a Neuro-Developmental Treatment frame of reference, because this will address his current level of development and build movement patterns that will lead to the parents' expected outcomes of intervention.

Another factor is the therapist's own skills and perspective. Though most occupational therapists have been taught a consistent body of knowledge, it may have been presented from different orientations and organized in different ways. For example, all professional educational programs base their content on the *Essentials & Guidelines for an Accredited Educational Program for the Occupational Therapist* (AOTA, 1991); however, this content may be taught using different orientations and emphasizing different areas. Some may focus more on specific treatment techniques, while others may accent the clinical reasoning process. Because of our individual differences in life experience and personality, material may be learned and interpreted differently. A therapist may identify a favorite frame of reference that he or she prefers to use. The last factor that may influence the choice of frame of reference is the setting in which services are being provided. For example, some frames of reference may not be able to be implemented within a home-based setting, a school-based setting, a community setting, or a hospital. While all of the factors mentioned may influence the choice of a frame of reference, the individual's needs should be given primary consideration.

It is important to keep in mind that the therapist still has merely a preliminary picture of the client's abilities, areas of difficulty, and needs. Once the therapist chooses his or her frame of reference or treatment approach for the client, the evaluation process continues. There needs to be a clear-cut relationship between the approach chosen and the assessments to be used. Again, the frame of reference will be used in this chapter to present the relationship between theory and evaluation. Since frame of reference has become an acceptable vehicle for organizing theoretical material and translating it into practice, the selection of the frame of reference determines which assessment tools are most appropriate. The frame of reference provides a linking structure between theory and practice (Kramer & Hinojosa, 1993; Hinojosa, Kramer, & Pratt, 1996).

A frame of reference draws from one or more theories to provide a basis for what will occur throughout the intervention process. Based on the theoretical information, the frame of reference presents specific behaviors or physical signs that are considered functional and specific behaviors that denote dysfunction (Mosey, 1992). Assessment tools are then chosen that will identify the presence of both functional and dysfunctional behaviors, as described within the theoretical base. Sometimes the frame of reference recommends specific tools. At other times, the behaviors or physical signs are clearly described, and it is left up to the therapist to determine which tool will best be able to identify the physical signs or behaviors. The theories that underlie the assessment tools need to be congruent with the theoretical information that formulates the treatment approach.

Evaluations are affected by philosophy in two ways: First, the philosophy of the profession guides the selection, interpretation, and administration of the tools; and second, many evaluation tools are themselves based on a philosophical perspective. The difficulty for occupational therapists is to achieve congruence between the tools that are used and the philosophies themselves. Are we constrained by the tools that currently exist, and do these really satisfy our domains of concerns and our areas of interest? People sometimes use tests because they are valued by other disciplines. They do not use the tests in the manner intended, because the tests do not adequately fit in with their own philosophies.

Clinical Reasoning in Evaluation

The majority of studies on the clinical reasoning process in occupational therapy have been published during the past 20 years. Schon (1983) describes the automatic responses of professionals as reflection-in-action. This reflection is described as an automatic process, where a practitioner thinks about a current situation that may be somewhat unusual, puts it into the context of previous similar situations, and then acts in a manner that will result in a better understanding of the issue as a whole. Rogers (1983) viewed clinical reasoning as containing dimensions of ethics, art, and science. She proposed that our reasoning process should follow the basic questions that the therapist is trying to answer in the clinical process.

Studies of clinical reasoning in occupational therapy have described the "therapist with the three-track mind" (Fleming, 1991, p. 1,007). These three tracks are procedural reasoning, interactive reasoning, and conditional reasoning. Procedural reasoning describes when the therapist focuses on the disease or disability and makes decisions on procedures and intervention activities based on this focus. Interactive reasoning requires the therapist to view the patient as an individual, rather than according to a diagnostic category. This usually takes place when the therapist is directly involved with the client. Conditional reasoning is the most complex level of this clinical reasoning process, requiring the therapist to understanding the diagnostic condition in its totality, as well as its effect on the individual, understanding how the condition can change, and engaging the individual as an active participant, determining the goals and expected outcomes of the intervention process. This phase of the reasoning process involves imagining and projecting expected outcomes as well as integrating all three types of reasoning (Fleming 1991,

1994). The process of evaluation requires interactive reasoning, at the very least, while conditional reasoning would be an essential component of the intervention planning process. Rogers and Holm (1991) referred to the sequence of decisions during the assessment process as "diagnostic reasoning" and viewed this as only one component of the clinical reasoning process.

Rogers and Masagatani (1982) looked at the clinical reasoning of occupational therapists during the initial assessment of individuals with physical disabilities. A qualitative method was used with data gathered through observations and interviews. Emerging themes were having compassion for the client and establishing a positive relationship. For the therapist, this led to intermingling the evaluation process with intervention. The development of an understanding of the client also appeared to be important. Therapists viewed themselves as being active and sensitive, but found it difficult to describe their thought processes, describing what they had done instead of the thought processes guiding their decisions.

A study examining the initial evaluation in psychosocial occupational therapy was done by Barris (1987), who noted that the therapist's treatment orientation did not appear to influence assessment, while the hospital setting appeared to be a major influence. The occupational therapy department in this setting chose the assessment to be used, leading to a more routinized assessment, rather than one that was tailored to the client, though therapists tended to rely more on information that they themselves had gathered, rather than on the medical chart.

Therapists have described the evaluation process as similar to solving a puzzle, where one piece of information can change one's whole view of the client and can lead to the need for different areas of exploration. It is a continuously reflective process, in which the therapist is using each piece of information to guide his or her actions and subsequent decisions. This process is benefitted by prior learning and experiences (Kramer, 1993).

Ideally, clinical reasoning during the evaluation process should combine the therapist's knowledge of the principles and theories of occupational therapy, and his or her prior experiences, with an understanding of the individual being evaluated and knowledge of the client's diagnosis or condition. This will allow the therapist to choose an appropriate frame of reference based on an adequate screening, which will guide the evaluation further by suggesting various assessments, as well as areas to be explored.

Summary

Occupational therapy is based in philosophy; therefore, the process of evaluation has a strong philosophical basis, and assessments combine a philosophical basis with a theoretical orientation. In choosing assessments, therapists need to be aware of the theoretical orientation of the assessment, as well as its consistency with the philosophy of occupational therapy. The choice of assessment tools has to be consistent with the needs of the individual and the frame of reference that the therapist will use with the client. The evaluation process is complex and requires continuous clinical reasoning, so that the therapist can adequately identify the needs and concerns of the client and the areas that require intervention.

References

American Occupational Therapy Association. (1991). *Essentials & guidelines for an accredited educational program for the occupational therapist.* Bethesda, MD: Author.

American Occupational Therapy Association. (1994). Uniform terminology for occupational therapy (3rd ed.). *American Journal of Occupational Therapy, 48,* 1047–1054.

Ayres, A. J. (1976, March). Clinical observations of neuromuscular integration. Administration of the Southern California Sensory Integration Tests, Certification Course. Conference sponsored by the Center for the Study of Sensory Integrative Dysfunction, held at Valhalla, NY.

Barris, R. (1987). Clinical reasoning in psychosocial occupational therapy. *Occupational Therapy Journal of Research, 7,* 147–162.

Bruininks, R. (1978). *Bruininks-Oseretsky test of motor proficiency.* Circle Pines, MN: American Guidance Service.

Bruce, M. A., & Borg, B. (1987). *Frames of reference in psychosocial occupational therapy.* Thorofare, NJ: Slack.

Christiansen, C. (1991). Occupational therapy: Intervention for life performance. In C. Christiansen & C. Baum (Eds.), *Occupational therapy: Overcoming human performance deficits* (pp. 3–43). Thorofare, NJ: Slack.

Collier, T. (1991). The screening process. In W. Dunn (Ed.), *Pediatric occupational therapy: Facilitating effective service provision* (pp. 11–33). Thorofare, NJ: Slack.

Farber, S.D. (1982). Neurorehabilitation evaluation concepts. In S.D. Farber (Ed.), *Neurorehabilitation: A multisensory approach* (pp. 107–114). Philadelphia: W.B. Saunders.

Frankenberg, W.K., Dodds, J., Archer, P., Bresnick, B., Maschka, P., Edelman, N., & Shapiro, H. (1991). *The Denver II Developmental Screening Test.* Denver, CO: Denver Developmental Materials.

Fleming, M.H. (1994). The therapist with the three-track mind. In C. Mattingly & M.H. Fleming (Eds.), *Clinical reasoning: Forms of inquiry in a therapeutic practice* (pp. 119–136). Philadelphia, PA: F.A. Davis.

Fleming, M.H. (1991). The therapist with the three-track mind. *American Journal of Occupational Therapy, 45,* 1007–1014.

Hinojosa, J., & Kramer, P. (1996). Integrating children with disabilities into family play. In L.D. Parham & L.S. Fazio (Eds.), *Play in occupational therapy for children* (pp. 159–170). Chicago, IL: Mosby.

Hinojosa, J., Kramer, P., & Pratt, P. N. (1996). Foundations of practice: Developmental principles, theories, and frame of reference. In J. Case-Smith, A.S. Allen, & P.N. Pratt (eds.), *Occupational therapy for children* (3rd ed.) (pp. 25–45). Chicago, IL: Mosby.

Jette, A. M., Davis, A. R., Cleary, P. D., Calkins, D.R., Rubenstein, L.V., Fink, A., Rosecroft, S., Young, R.T., Brook, R.H., & Delbanco, T.L. (1986). The functional status questionnaire: Reliability and validity when used in primary care. *Journal of General Internal Medicine, 1,* 143–149.

Keilhofner, G. (1992). *Conceptual foundations of occupational therapy.* Philadelphia, PA: F.A. Davis.

Kramer, P. (1993). *Pediatric occupational therapist's views of their procedures and practices when evaluating children.* Unpublished doctoral dissertation, New York University, NY.

Kramer, P., & Hinojosa, J. (1993). Structure of the frame of reference. In P. Kramer & J. Hinojosa (Eds.), *Frame of reference in pediatric occupational therapy* (pp. 37–48). Baltimore, MD: Williams & Wilkins.

Matsutsuyu, J. (1969). The interest checklist. *American Journal of Occupational Therapy, 23,* 323–328.

Moorehead, L.M. (1969). The occupational history. *American Journal of Occupational Therapy, 23,* 329–336.

Mosey, A.C. (1970). *Three frames of reference for mental health.* Thorofare, NJ: Slack.

Mosey, A.C. (1981). *Occupational therapy: Configuration of a profession.* New York: Raven Press.

Mosey, A.C. (1986). *Psychosocial components of occupational therapy.* New York: Raven Press.

Mosey, A.C. (1992). *Applied scientific inquiry in the health professions: An epistemological orientation.* Bethesda, MD. American Occupational Therapy Association.

Mosey, A.C. (1996). *Applied scientific inquiry in the health professions: An epistemological orientation* (2nd ed.). Bethesda, MD: American Occupational Therapy Association.

Reed, K.L., & Sanderson, S.N. (1992). *Concepts of occupational therapy* (3rd ed). Baltimore, MD: Williams & Wilkins.

Rogers, J. (1983). Clinical reasoning: The ethics, science and art. *American Journal of Occupational Therapy, 37,* 601–616.

Rogers, J., & Hold, M.B. (1991). Occupational therapy diagnostic reasoning: A component of clinical reasoning. *American Journal of Occupational Therapy, 45,* 1045–1053.

Rogers, J., & Masagatani, G. (1982). Clinical reasoning of occupational therapists during the initial assessment of physically disabled patients. *Occupational Therapy Journal of Research, 2,* 195–219.

Schon, D. (1983). *The reflective practitioner: How professionals think in action.* New York: Basic Books.

Stewart, K. B. (1996). Occupational therapy assessment in pediatrics: Purposes, process, and methods of evaluation. In J. Case-Smith, A.S. Allen, & P.N. Pratt (Eds.), *Occupational therapy for children* (3rd ed.) (pp. 165–199). St. Louis: Mosby.

3 Uniform Terminology and its Application to Occupational Therapy Evaluation

Cathy Dolhi, OTR/L
Mary Lou Leibold, MS, OTRL/L

Overview

This chapter reviews the development and application of *Uniform Terminology* to occupational therapy practice and specifically illustrates its use as a valuable tool in the evaluation process. It includes a discussion of the domain of concern for occupational therapy, with examples to illustrate how to apply *Uniform Terminology* in day-to-day practice. Through the presentation of case examples, the relationship of *Uniform Terminology* to the occupational therapy evaluation process is illustrated.

Introduction

A screening is completed as the initial step in the course of establishing a plan of treatment for the individual referred for occupational therapy. The evaluation is an ongoing process whereby the occupational therapy practitioner gathers all the vital information needed to determine a plan of intervention. The completeness and accuracy of the evaluation are crucial as they set the basis for the type of intervention that the individual will receive. The evaluation

29

must be holistic and sufficiently encompassing to clearly delineate areas where the therapist may assist the individual by identifying strengths and weaknesses. The evaluation should consider these strengths and weaknesses within the context of the individual's goals, values, habits, and life in general. Upon determining areas of need, the occupational therapist, in collaboration with the individual and possibly significant others, can construct a plan to address issues that will enhance the individual's functional performance abilities. An important resource available to occupational therapy personnel for guiding the evaluation process is *Uniform Terminology for Occupational Therapy* (3rd ed.) (AOTA, 1994).

Background of *Uniform Terminology*

In response to the Medicare and Medicaid Anti-Fraud and Abuse Amendments (Public Law 95-142) passed in October 1977, which required health care facilities to establish a uniform reporting system, AOTA developed the *Occupational Therapy Output Reporting System* and the *Uniform Terminology System for Reporting Occupational Therapy Services* (AOTA, 1979). Although the uniform reporting system was not adopted by the Department of Health and Human Services, the *Uniform Terminology* section was used extensively by occupational therapy practitioners as a glossary to ensure consistency in definitions.

The *Uniform Terminology* document was revised in 1989 to become current with changes in practice and was expanded to encompass the scope of practice (AOTA, 1989). Modifications included recategorization and refining of content, and the inclusion of more precise definitions. In 1994, the document was again revised, with another recategorization of content and the incorporation of contextual aspects of performance. This third edition was intended to define the domain of concern of occupational therapy practice (AOTA, 1994).

Uniform Terminology (3rd ed.) (Appendix B) defines three parameters of occupational therapy's domain of concern: *performance areas, performance components,* and *performance contexts.* Outlining the details and definitions in each of these areas is of tremendous importance to the occupational therapy profession for a number of reasons. First, it creates a guide for therapists to reference throughout the evaluation process and course of intervention. Second, it guides the therapist to think holistically, considering the "entire person," rather than honing in on a medical diagnosis or a single performance deficit. Third, it provides a common ground of understanding and facilitates consistency among occupational therapy practitioners, academicians, researchers, and students. Finally, *Uniform Terminology* provides a framework for explaining occupational therapy to others, including clients, significant others, third-party payers, and other professionals.

PERFORMANCE AREAS

The performance areas are broad categories that consist of activities that are typically performed throughout the course of an individual's daily life. Within the context of *Uniform Terminology,* these areas encompass the things that individuals want or need to do and include activities of daily living, work and productive activities, and play or leisure activities. The importance of these performance areas to the individual will differ greatly depending on the life roles of the person. Roles are defined as "distinctive positions in society, each having a defined status, and specific expectations for behavior" (Christiansen, 1991, p. 28). Common examples of roles might include student, parent, or worker.

Determining an individual's need and desire to perform specific role-related activities outlined in the performance areas is a logical first step of the occupational therapy evaluation. For example, "grooming" may be of major importance to the adolescent female and much less important to the older client, whereas "medication routine" may be vital to the older person and a nonissue to the adolescent. Therefore, goals for independence in grooming may be identified by the adolescent as highly important. Areas to be addressed can be identified through interviews with the client and significant others, chart review, review of diagnostic implications, and direct observation of the individual's ability to perform the identified activities.

Many different subcategories of the three performance areas are included in the *Uniform Terminology* document, and each is operationally defined. The therapist should consider each area for its appropriateness to the individual and evaluate it accordingly. This list of subcategories can be used as a checklist and is quite valuable, as it prompts the therapist to consider each area in totality. Skillful evaluation requires the therapist to uncover the person's prior occupations and activities and analyze how those have been affected by illness, injury, or developmental problems. Intervention planning further requires clarification of the individual's expectations for the future and motivation for change. Throughout this evaluation and planning process, all relevant areas identified in *Uniform Terminology* should be included; however, the individual and an understanding of his or her life shall determine what will be involved in intervention. The therapist may use questions such as, "What did a typical day or week look like for you?" or "How were your weekends different from your weekdays?" to help understand the person's prior occupations. For example, a client may say, "Oh honey, my wife does all the cooking; I don't need this." Upon further investigation, the therapist may learn that the client is actually alone during the day and must prepare a light lunch for himself. Thus, thoughtful and tactful interview questions, along with selected activities, can be used to paint the client's occupational profile and determine which performance areas must be addressed.

Case Example

ADDRESSING PERFORMANCE AREAS

Mrs. Jones is a 77-year-old woman who fell, fractured her right hip, and had a total hip replacement. She is an inpatient in a rehabilitation unit and is referred to the occupational therapy department for evaluation and treatment. The diagnostic implications of "total hip replacement" immediately alert the therapist to orthopedic precautions that must be followed. These include lower extremity range of motion and strength limitations, weight-bearing restrictions, and the potential for developing deep venous thrombosis, all of which affect the client's mobility status. Upon interviewing Mrs. Jones, the occupational therapist learns that prior to fracturing her hip, Mrs. Jones, a retired department store clerk, lived alone in her own home. In addition to performing her activities of daily living and home management tasks independently, Mrs. Jones used public transportation for shopping, regularly attended a local senior citizens' center, and participated in church-related activities. Based on a review of the chart and discussions with Mrs. Jones, the therapist finds that Mrs. Jones has two supportive children who live out of town, both of whom are willing to have their mother move in with them if she is unable to live alone. ■

These few pieces of information provide the therapist with a "snapshot" of Mrs. Jones' premorbid occupational roles and discharge options. Mrs. Jones' goal is to return to her own home and resume those activities in which she participated prior to her hip fracture. It is the therapist's responsibility now to determine Mrs. Jones' skill level with regard to each of the performance areas, activities of daily living, productive living and work, and play and leisure, focusing particularly on those that have been identified as important to her.

This step of the evaluation begins with an interview focusing on self-care activities such as dressing and bathing. This is verified via a bedside session and clinical simulation of self-care activities. A thorough understanding of Mrs. Jones' abilities is the area of self-care will help to determine her discharge plan and thus will influence the evaluation of other performance areas. As Mrs. Jones progresses, further assessments related to home, community-based work, and productive and leisure activities are completed as appropriate. The primary objective of the interpretation is to determine whether Mrs. Jones would be able to return to her home and live independently, performing those life functions that are important to her, or whether she would need to modify her plans and consider living with one of her children.

In addition to observation and interview, the therapist should consider standardized assessment tools designed to evaluate effectiveness within each performance area. While the therapist's choice of tools will depend on needs of the client and the service delivery model, as well as the therapist's theoretical orientation, therapists are encouraged to incorporate valid and reliable measures of performance (see chapters 5, 6, 7). If it is determined that there are limitations in a particular performance area for the client, the therapist then examines the performance components and performance contexts.

PERFORMANCE COMPONENTS

The performance components are the underlying abilities that are required for an individual to participate in a given performance area. The performance components are categorized as sensorimotor components, cognitive integration and cognitive components, and psychosocial skills and psychological components. An occupational therapist may address a performance component in two ways. First, when a therapist has information that a specific deficit exists in a performance component, he or she may directly evaluate and plan interventions related to the specific performance component. Second, when a person is not independent in one or more of the performance areas, the therapist may question why this is occurring. The therapist then begins a systematic evaluation of each performance component and its subcomponent aspects. For example, the therapist asks, is it a sensorimotor problem (e.g., reduced strength or sensation), a cognitive deficit (e.g., decreased attention span or memory), or a psychosocial or psychological issue (e.g., impaired self-concept or inadequate coping skills) that is impeding function?

The components of a particular activity may be identified initially via activity analysis. The *Uniform Terminology Grid* presented in *Uniform Terminology for Occupational Therapy* (3rd ed.) *Application to Practice* (Appendix C) provides one such activity analysis tool designed to help the therapist relate performance components and performance contexts to performance areas. By using the grids as a reference, the therapist is prompted to be systematically comprehensive about considering the potential impact of each element on the performance areas.

Consider the example of Mrs. Jones. Following the introductory interview and a bedside treatment session, the therapist confirmed that Mrs. Jones needed maximum assistance to complete lower body dressing. The therapist locates "dressing" on the horizontal axis of the grid and follows the column down the vertical axis to determine which of the performance component(s) contributes to Mrs. Jones' inability to perform lower body dressing independently. Thorough consideration of the various possibilities leads the therapist to the conclusion that deficits in the sensorimotor components of range of motion, strength, endurance, and activity tolerance directly correlate with

Mrs. Jones' difficulty with lower body dressing. In addition, the acuity of Mrs. Jones' medical condition influences her ability to manage the activity, when considered as a temporal feature within performance contexts.

Likewise, having identified a deficit in one of the performance components, the therapist may begin on the vertical axis and move horizontally across the grid to determine whether the component has an impact on the performance areas relevant to the client. For example, when considering the diagnostic implications of "total hip replacement," the therapist will acknowledge the likelihood of deficits in lower extremity range of motion and strength. Locating these performance components on the *Uniform Terminology Grid* and simultaneously considering each performance area in relation to those components will ensure that the therapist has fully considered the potential impact of the performance component deficit on the performance areas.

By considering each performance area and the relatedness of the performance components and contextual factors, the therapist can generate a graphical representation of the client's performance deficits. This can serve as a "blueprint" for the occupational therapy treatment plan and can help the therapist, client, and others involved in the client's care to visually perceive how the performance areas, performance components, and contextual factors are interrelated.

Having determined the preliminary reasons for performance deficits, the therapist will now begin to identify an appropriate frame of reference and the assessment tools that will enable him or her to more specifically pinpoint performance assets and liabilities. These may include sensorimotor assessments that determine visual perceptual skills, range of motion, and manual muscle testing, or gross/fine motor coordination assessments; cognitive assessment tools designed to assess short-term memory, sequencing, attention span, or problem-solving capabilities; or assessment instruments that provide insight into the client's self-concept, interpersonal skills, or time-management adeptness. Understanding the results of these "component-oriented" evaluations will help to identify the source of the performance problem and the focus for eventual intervention.

Case Example

ADDRESSING PERFORMANCE COMPONENTS

The case of Mrs. Jones, considered previously with a focus on the performance areas could also be explored with a focus on performance components. The therapist determines, upon interview and clinical observation, that Mrs. Jones requires assistance with lower body bathing and dressing due to sensorimotor deficits in the areas of lower extremity range of motion, strength, and endurance. The same components contribute to deficits in functional mobility, especially bed mobility, transfers, and functional ambulation, as well as toilet hygiene. In addition, the therapist notes that Mrs. Jones has strengths in the cognitive, psychosocial and psychological component areas, as she is able to quickly incorporate and apply compensatory techniques taught to her (e.g., problem solving, learning, generalization). Also, she views the ability to perform tasks without assistance as a priority (e.g., values, self-concept, coping skills, and self-control), which will positively influence her rehabilitation. By working on her sensorimotor deficits and functional mobility, Mrs. Jones may be able to achieve her goal of independent living. The *Uniform Terminology Grid* is also a valuable tool for prompting the therapist to consider the client's areas of strength and incorporating them into the ensuing treatment plan. ∎

PERFORMANCE CONTEXTS

The context in which an individual performs a particular activity has significant influence on his or her ability to engage successfully in the performance area. Performance contexts are defined by *Uniform Terminology* as "situations or factors that influence an individual's engagement in desired and/or required performance areas" (AOTA, 1994, p. 1047). Performance contexts consist of temporal and environmental aspects. Temporal features are divided into chronological age, developmental age, place in the lifecycle, and disability status. Environmental considerations are divided into physical, social, and cultural. When each of these aspects is considered in relation to the individual, the uniqueness of each person becomes apparent. Identifying that individuality is the key to pinpointing important roles and related areas of performance areas for each person. Then, based on all the information, the plan of intervention is determined.

For example, if one considers the performance area of "socialization" in isolation, the definition refers to "accessing opportunities and interacting with other people in appropriate contextual and cultural ways to meet emotional and physical needs" (AOTA, 1994, p. 1051). However, the implications for "socialization" change dramatically when one adds the contextual considerations. Consider the implications of "socialization" for a spinal-cord-injured adolescent living at home with his parents, as opposed to those associated with a senior citizen with a chronic disability residing in a long-term-care facility. The contextual factors (e.g., age, place in the lifecycle, social and cultural elements, and physical environment) of these two cases force the therapist to consider different scenarios regarding "socialization." Therefore, the focus of the occupational therapy evaluation and intervention would be different in these two cases, because of the contextual variations. A number of assessment tools is available to determine environmental impact on performance (Letts, Law, Rigby, Cooper, Stewart, & Strong, 1994). Although fewer tools are available to deal with other contextual factors (Dunn, Brown, & McGuigan, 1994), the therapist can gain much through observation and interview.

Case Example

ADDRESSING PERFORMANCE CONTEXT

Again returning to the case of Mrs. Jones, the therapist must consider the implications of her age, place in the lifecycle, and the fact that in the absence of other complicating medical conditions, the restrictions related to the acuteness of her injury will likely be temporary. Likewise, the therapist needs to determine the environmental aspects that will positively or negatively affect her potential functional capacity after discharge from the rehabilitation setting. For Mrs. Jones, these considerations will include the fact that her bed and bathroom are located on the second floor of her home, but, if necessary, temporary accommodations could be set up on the first floor for her safety and convenience. In addition, she has a reliable support system of family and friends who have expressed a desire and ability to provide short-term assistance. ∎

Illustrating the Use of Uniform Terminology

The following case examples are provided to further illustrate how *Uniform Terminology* can be used as a framework for evaluation. Each example delineates how *Uniform Terminology* can be used during the screening and evaluation of clients. Each case example is organized by including all three parameters of occupational therapy's domain of concern and addressing the one that appears most influential in each case first. However, they are examined in different orders and with various emphasis. The unique features of each case will help to illustrate the rationale for the manner in which the evaluation process was approached.

Case Example

MR. BROWN—PERFORMANCE CONTEXT/PERFORMANCE AREAS/PERFORMANCE COMPONENTS

Mr. Brown is a 55-year-old successful business executive. He was on the road, working long hours Monday through Friday, living in hotels and eating all of his meals in restaurants. He returned home to spend relaxing leisurely weekends with his wife, who also had a prestigious job in business and worked long hours during the week. She did not travel but stayed alone at their home during the week. She ate most of her meals as "take-out" from restaurants and had hired help for most home management activities (e.g., cleaning, laundry, lawn care).

Mr. Brown had a subarachnoid hemorrhage, was admitted to an inpatient rehabilitation center, and was referred to occupational therapy and later followed through as an outpatient. After 2 weeks of an inpatient stay, activities of daily living were performed with moderate assistance to modified independence. Home management and leisure activities were of great interest to Mr. Brown, but he had not spent much time pursuing them for many years, due to his busy work life.

With regard to performance contexts, important considerations for this client were that he had planned on retiring in the next couple of years, that the residual effects of a subarachnoid hemorrhage are typically permanent, and that he had a very supportive wife and circle of friends. He was able to retire early due to his disability and expressed interest in taking on more home management tasks. Through delicate yet frank discussions among Mr. and Mrs. Brown and his therapist, it was determined that he would focus his attention on assuming different home responsibilities and taking on new life roles. Mr. Brown and his wife decided that he could attempt to take on home management roles, while the wife would continue to work outside the home. Occupational therapy intervention then focused on performance components that would strengthen his abilities in the performance areas of independence in activities of daily living and home management, both in inpatient and outpatient care. The context of Mr. Brown's age, previous life role, and current interests, combined with the understanding of Mrs. Brown and her willingness to adjust to differing roles, sets the stage for this evaluation and intervention.

Performance components were considered next. Mild deficits were noted in perceptual processing and cognitive components such as memory and personal organization. These, along with deficits in his interpersonal skills, including relating to others, especially in group situations, were frustrating to Mr. Brown, as he realized his decreased functional abilities. From a physical standpoint, both upper extremities were functional for his daily living skills, and he ambulated with minimal supervision and only an occasional loss of balance. Evaluating Mr. Brown's skills following his occupational therapy intervention, it was found that these deficit areas would not interfere with Mr. Brown's performance in his newly acquired role.

This illustration is intended to demonstrate the challenge when a person is unable to return to a performance area or primary life role, and how his performance context, including his age and environment, can contribute to a successful intervention. In Mr. Brown's case, performance contexts were addressed first. Important considerations were that he was nearing retirement, the effects of the subarachnoid hemorrhage were estimated to be longstanding and prohibitive of the client returning to work in the near future, and the willingness of the wife to be involved in her husband's rehabilitation care plan and eventual role reversal with him. Second, performance areas were addressed, and goals revolving around enhancing his independence in activities of daily living and home management were addressed to facilitate the role reversal with his wife. Third, performance components were addressed, and compensatory techniques for perceptual deficits were used. By systematically looking at performance contexts, performance components, and performance areas, the therapist has a guide to managing cases that may otherwise be much more difficult. In this case, Mr. Brown's age, his ability to retire, and his wife's willingness to engage in some role changes allowed Mr. Brown to continue with a productive life. ■

Case Example

LISA—PERFORMANCE COMPONENTS/PERFORMANCE AREAS/PERFORMANCE CONTEXT

Lisa is a 17-year-old who has been in a persistent vegetative state for 6 months following a car accident. Her parents weighed the options for long-term placement and decided to take her home to live with them and her 15-year-old sister. Prior to her accident, Lisa was a senior in high school and was very active in sports, socializing with her friends and working part-time as a waitress to earn money for college.

Upon discharge to her home, occupational therapy was ordered. The evaluation done by the home-based therapist showed that Lisa had severe deficits in many performance components. She responded only to pain; she demonstrated highly increased flexor tone throughout her body; she showed no purposeful movement; and she did not respond to environmental stimuli. Because of these deficits in performance components, Lisa was completely dependent in all performance areas of activities of daily living, work and productive activities, and play or leisure.

Contextually, the client was early in her life cycle. Undoubtedly, Lisa would have a chronic disability; however, the extent was not truly known.

Finally, Lisa had a supportive and available family, which was very willing to be involved with her care.

In this case, performance components were evaluated first, because of the very low-level functioning of the client, so as to determine the potential for engagement in performance areas in the future. Contextual components were significant, as the client was taken home by the family, which had no medical background. Intervention focused on family training in certain therapeutic strategies, highlighting sensorimotor components, maximizing the physical and social environment, as well as providing basic skills in caring for Lisa. Concurrently, the therapist worked on providing stimulation for Lisa, in order to obtain sensory responses, and guiding her through some basic activities of daily living. As therapy progressed, Lisa's responses and subsequent possible changes would determine whether the intervention would move into addressing performance areas more directly. At the same time, the therapist would apprize the family of the need to adapt or change the physical and social environment to assist in Lisa's continued recovery. ■

Case Example

MR. GREEN—PERFORMANCE AREAS/PERFORMANCE CONTEXT/PERFORMANCE COMPONENTS

Mr. Green recently became a resident of a long-term-care facility, after hospitalization from a stroke. He is 85 years old and had previously lived with his wife of the same age. Prior to the stroke, he placed a high degree of value on socialization and remaining active with other people. He loved to converse with others, listen to music, sing church hymns, and play cards. Mrs. Green determined that she would not be able to physically provide all the help that her husband would need, and a long-term-care facility close to their home was selected.

Occupational therapy was ordered for the client at the long-term-care facility. Evaluation of performance areas showed that Mr. Green needed assistance with activities of daily living and valued independence in that area. He required moderate assistance with grooming, dressing, and feeding/eating. He required maximum assistance with bathing, toilet hygiene, medication routine, health maintenance, and community mobility. Mr. Green was dependent in home management activities; however, these activities were completed for him in the context of the long-term-care facility.

Important aspects of performance contexts for Mr. Green are that he is elderly and has residuals from a stroke that are potentially chronic.

The physical environment of the long-term-care facility is positive, as it is wheelchair accessible and supports Mr. Green's highest level of functional performance. Caregivers are available to provide assistance as needed. His wife loves him dearly but is simply unable to physically care for him in their home, due to her age and the inaccessibility of the home.

From a performance component standpoint, Mr. Green showed deficits in the cognitive areas that included reduced orientation, attention span, ability to initiate and sequence an activity, as well as poor problem-solving skills. His left upper extremity was nonfunctional, with decreased passive range of motion in shoulder flexion and abduction, one-half breadth finger subluxation, pain at the shoulder, and no active movement. Multiple perceptual problems were identified. His unsupported sitting and standing balance are fair, and he is nonambulatory. He requires maximum assistance to negotiate a wheelchair around the facility.

In this case, we looked at Mr. Green holistically by first addressing performance areas, then the performance context and performance components. The findings for this client suggest that the long-term-care environment, at this time, best suits the needs of both Mr. and Mrs. Green. The therapist develops a plan of intervention focusing on those skills that are most important to Mr. Green. These include being able to use the telephone so that he may keep in close contact with his wife, and being functionally mobile around the facility in his wheelchair so that he may go where he likes. His priorities also include being independent with bathing and grooming as well as eating/feeding, so that he is comfortable in a group setting and, especially when his wife comes to visit, being able to participate in the group sing-a-long provided by the staff of the facility and being able to socialize with other residents, especially through conservation and playing cards. By addressing these areas, the therapist can help Mr. Green, not only with specific performance components, but ultimately with the performance areas of activities of daily living, and play or leisure activities that are so important to him. ∎

Case Example

JEFF—PERFORMANCE AREAS/PERFORMANCE COMPONENTS/PERFORMANCE CONTEXT

Jeff is a 38-year-old with a long history of schizophrenia, who has been living alone in his own apartment. He has been in and out of the hospital many times over the past 8 months, for relapses related to his mental health condition. When Jeff maintains an appropriate medication regime, keeping his schizophrenia under control, he works at a cable company as an installer. He also goes to the gym three times a week and visits his niece and nephew on a weekly basis. Jeff has recently been admitted to the inpatient psychiatric unit of a local hospital, due to an increasing inability to care for himself, locking himself in his house, and not reporting to work. He has been referred to occupational therapy for evaluation and treatment.

When Jeff enters the clinic area, the therapist notes that his hair is uncombed, his clothes are dirty, and he is in need of a shower. Upon talking with him, the therapist verifies that Jeff has been withdrawn, not reporting to work, and has been indifferent about performing basic self-care and home management activities. Utilizing the *Uniform Technology Grid,* the therapist discusses with Jeff his recent effectiveness in each of the performance areas, and determines whether or not a decline has occurred. The therapist looks at each performance area in question and moves vertically down each column to consider the impact of the various performance components. This process enables the therapist to systematically identify potential areas of deficit and strengths. Standardized evaluations in the areas of cognition, psychosocial skills, and psychological components are used to identify strengths and weakness in these performance components. The assessment results confirm the therapist's initial hypothesis that Jeff has difficulty with the cognitive performance components related to initiating activity, maintaining his attention for greater than 10 minutes, implementing problem-solving strategies, sequencing, categorization, and generalization. Jeff also is unable to identify activities or things that are important to him, has difficulty expressing himself, and, as evidenced by his isolating behavior, is lacking in adequate coping skills. Jeff is most aware of his recent functional decline and considers himself to be a "bad person" because of it.

Consideration of the contextual factors in relation to the performance areas (in the same manner as previously described) provides the therapist with valuable information that must be regarded in Jeff's case. Jeff desperately wants to return to his apartment and his job. Given his relatively young age and the chronic nature of his schizophrenia, it is important that he learn and consistently implement more effective strategies for ensuring his mental health and safety. Based on his frequent hospital admission since living alone, the therapist questions whether that living environment is adequate for Jeff's needs at the present time.

By considering this information holistically, Jeff and the therapist can begin to develop an intervention program that will target those areas in which he is experiencing performance breakdown. It may be in Jeff's best interest to move temporarily to a more structured environment (personal care or other supervised setting) where he can practice implementing strategies that will ultimately support his ability to live independently in the future.

This case attends to performance areas initially, since deficits in these areas are the primary reason for Jeff's current hospitalization. Evaluation of the performance components and contextual factors and how they impact Jeff's ability to successfully function in the community are considered as the next step with intervention strategies targeted toward those areas that will enhance his effectiveness in the performance areas. ∎

Case Example

GINA—PERFORMANCE COMPONENTS/PERFORMANCE CONTEXT/PERFORMANCE AREAS

Seven-year-old Gina has been referred to occupational therapy as part of her Individual Education Plan (IEP) for second grade. Following a difficult year in first grade, Gina was diagnosed with attention deficit disorder (ADD). As reported in the referral information and preevaluation questionnaire that included categories of behavioral characteristics, her classroom teacher and her mother indicate that Gina tends to be clumsy, has poor handwriting skills, frequently does not wait for her turn, loses papers and school supplies, and is inclined to play alone rather than with other children. The therapist highlights the areas of concern, as identified by the records, the teacher, and Gina's mother, on the *Uniform Terminology Grid* and uses this as a starting place for the occupational therapy evaluation. With the diagnostic implications of ADD and apparent performance deficits in the areas of activities of daily living (e.g., socialization, writing, and functional mobility), work and productive activities (i.e., educational activities), and play/leisure activities (i.e., play exploration and performance), the therapist is equipped with a basic understanding of areas of concern for Gina.

Given Gina's age and the diffuse nature of deficits associated with ADD, the therapist decides that it is most beneficial to present Gina with structured activities or assessment tools that will target the performance components in question. By dealing at the component level, the therapist can clearly identify the deficits that Gina is experiencing and can subsequently, by observation and/or interview with the classroom teacher and mother, determine how those components affect the relevant performance areas.

In examining performance components, the therapist identifies deficits in the areas of sensory processing, perceptual, and motor skills. Additionally, Gina lacks skills in all of the cognitive components with the exception of level of arousal and orientation and demonstrates significant deficits in the areas of social and self-management behaviors. Given her performance liabilities, school is a demanding environment for Gina.

Consideration of the performance contexts provides the therapist with additional information and insight. The fact that Gina is a child with limited life experience and has ADD, which can distort her perception of experiences, helps to build the framework for evaluation and intervention. Physical and social environmental characteristics will be critical in determining whether and how changes in the environment will affect Gina's ability to perform. The therapist intentionally manipulates the environment in which Gina is evaluated to determine how space, other people, and background noise affect her performance. These findings will influence subsequent treatment sessions and recommendations provided to the classroom teacher and mother. Furthermore, since this evaluation and intervention will take place at school, context and educational relevance will be especially important. The support, interest, and understanding of the teacher and mother are also contextual features that will assist in promoting successful carry-over.

In this example, consideration of the performance components initially is the preferred approach, since the therapist had been provided with referral information describing component deficits. The context of Gina's age and limited life experience, combined with the school setting, make it somewhat more complicated to deal initially at a performance area level. By looking at the components first, the therapist can then "back into" performance areas and gain confirmation related to Gina's performance from the teacher and mother. ∎

Case Example

JOAN—PERFORMANCE CONTEXTS/PERFORMANCE AREAS/PERFORMANCE COMPONENTS

Joan is a 29-year-old female who sustained a T-12 spinal cord injury 6 years ago. Since her injury, she has married and has resumed teaching fourth grade. Joan is now in the sixth month of her first pregnancy and has been referred to occupational therapy due to her increasing difficulty with managing her daily activities. Upon meeting her, the therapist learns that prior to her pregnancy, Joan was independent in all areas of activities of daily living, work, and leisure, and that her recent functional difficulties are directly related to her pregnancy.

Joan uses a lightweight wheelchair for mobility, has a wheelchair-accessible van, and resides with her husband in a two-story home that is equipped with a stairglide to the second floor, where the bedroom and bathroom are located. The couple's parents and siblings are supportive but live out of state and are unable to provide day-to-day assistance.

Joan notes that due to her increasing body weight, she is having difficulty with transfers, but that her husband is available to assist her in the morning and in the evening. She is also having difficulty managing her lower body bathing and dressing; is unable to reach into low cabinets and storage areas at home and at work; notes a moderate degree of upper extremity pain and fatigue related to propelling her wheelchair; and is exhausted at the end of her workday.

Physical examination reveals information about performance components. Joan's unsupported trunk balance is fair, since her center of gravity has been altered as a result of her pregnancy. She has good upper body strength and functional capabilities, but her activity tolerance is poor. She has no function in her lower extremities.

This case illustrates how influential performance context can be with regard to an individual's functional capability. Previously self-sufficient, the physical changes associated with her pregnancy have temporarily hampered Joan's ability to maintain her independence. Therefore, the therapist immediately acknowledges that it is contextual features that are the primary grounds for Joan's current condition. Knowing that the limitations are temporary in nature, the therapist explores other contextual issues to determine how they are affecting her. Being aware of the contextual framework in which Joan typically functions enables the therapist to examine how functional declines in the performance areas are related to impairments in the performance components. ■

Summary

In summary, *Uniform Terminology for Occupational Therapy* (3rd ed.) is a document created by the American Occupational Therapy Association for use by occupational therapy practitioners. It is a language that identifies the key areas to be addressed by occupational therapists with their clients and comprises performance areas, performance components, and performance contexts.

Performance areas are occupationally based and are made up of tasks that individuals need or want to perform, including activities of daily living, work and productive activities, and play or leisure activities. Performance components are the underlying skills that allow an individual to participate in a given performance area and include sensorimotor, cognitive, and psychosocial, plus psychological skills. For each individual, the performance components may either be strengths or weaknesses that support or impede performance. Performance contexts are the situations or factors that influence an individual's ability to perform. These include both temporal and environmental aspects and can be considered as an "umbrella" under which the performance components and performance areas are integrated.

The actual use of *Uniform Terminology* in clinical practice is flexible. Some therapists may choose to investigate performance areas first and assess the impact of the performance component and performance contextual factors subsequently. Others may choose to consider performance components and/ or performance contexts initially and then determine how those contribute to the individual's ability to participate within the performance areas. This can clearly be seen in the case examples cited in this chapter.

Factors that may influence the sequence in which areas are addressed include the client's medical or occupational diagnosis, the practice setting, the acuteness or chronic nature of the client's condition, the client's level of insight into the situation, and/or the therapist's theoretical orientation. Regardless of the order in which the performance areas, performance components, and performance contexts are considered, the primary value of utilizing *Uniform Terminology for Occupational Therapy* (3rd ed.) (AOTA, 1994) and the *Application of Uniform Terminology to Practice* (AOTA, 1994) Grid lies in the inherent design of the documents, which obliges the therapist to critically analyze and integrate the areas of concern for occupational therapy evaluation and subsequent intervention.

While the document is not prescriptive in nature, *Uniform Terminology* can be used as a tool to systematically guide the therapist through the evaluation process. This use of *Uniform Terminology* in a structured fashion promotes a holistic look at each client, facilitates completion of a comprehensive evaluation, and creates consistency among occupational therapy practitioners. It helps to target the areas of need and, ultimately, areas for intervention, as illustrated in the case studies.

References

American Occupational Therapy Association. (1979). *Occupational therapy output reporting system and uniform terminology system for reporting occupational therapy services.* Bethesda, MD: Author.

American Occupational Therapy Association. (1989). Uniform terminology for occupational therapy (2nd ed.). *American Journal of Occupational Therapy, 43,* 808–814.

American Occupational Therapy Association. (1994). Uniform terminology for occupational therapy (3rd ed.). *American Journal of Occupational Therapy, 48,* 1047–1054.

American Occupational Therapy Association. (1994). Application of uniform terminology to practice. *American Journal of Occupational Therapy, 48,* 1055–1059.

Christiansen, C. (1991). Occupational therapy: Intervention for life performance. In C. Christiansen & C. Baum (Eds.), *Occupational therapy: Overcoming human performance deficits* (pp. 3–43). Thorofare, NJ: Slack.

Dunn, W., Brown, C., & McGuigan, A. (1994). The ecology of human performance: A framework for considering the effect of context. *American Journal of Occupational Therapy, 48,* 595–607.

Letts, L., Law, M., Rigby, P., Cooper, B., Stewart, D., & Strong, S. (1994). Person-environment assessments in occupational therapy. *American Journal of Occupational Therapy, 48,* 608–618.

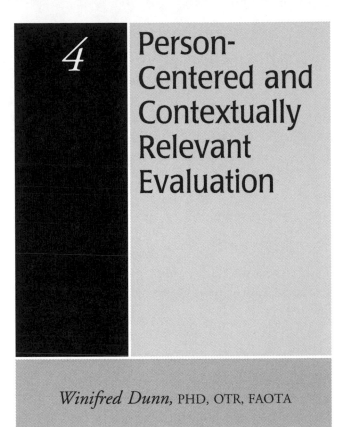

4 Person-Centered and Contextually Relevant Evaluation

Winifred Dunn, PHD, OTR, FAOTA

Overview

The first purpose of this chapter is to introduce the reader to the concept of person-centered evaluation and care, which requires professionals to shift their focus away from their own priorities and address the priorities of the individuals being served and their families. The second purpose of this chapter is to introduce a framework for evaluation of performance within appropriate contexts and to familiarize the reader with methods for constructing evaluation processes that include performance within the natural contexts. Finally, this chapter addresses how to use person-centered data in a contextually relevant manner.

Although most of the formal assessments available to occupational therapists evaluate the person's skills and abilities either as separate component skills or as part of task performance, these approaches neglect a critical source of information. A person's performance can be quite variable in different contexts. For example, an adolescent may have difficulty concentrating on school work when there are other students talking in the hall but may be perfectly able to screen out radio music to concentrate when studying. A gourmet cook will not be able to demonstrate advanced cooking skills in a primitive cabin in the woods. A young child may indeed be able to wash hands in the familiarity of the bathroom at home but may be confused about performing this task in the early childhood center. These examples demonstrate that performance can be context dependent; professionals run the risk of drawing incorrect conclusions when they fail to consider the impact of particular contexts as part of the data-gathering process.

Another critical but frequently overlooked aspect of quality evaluation is a consideration of the person's interests and needs. In person-centered care, professionals demonstrate awareness of and respect for what the individual and family being served wish to accomplish. This awareness of their wishes frames the entire evaluation process, so that the professional only considers strengths and barriers to the performance of those tasks that the individual and family have identified. This philosophy requires professionals to depart from traditional expert models of service, in which the professional directs the course of evaluation and planning based on his or her own best judgment about the situation.

Conducting Person-Centered Evaluations

Pollock (1993) describes several issues that arise when using traditional evaluation methods. First, she questions the appropriateness of professionals assigning performance scores to persons who are being evaluated; she suggests that only the person (and family, if appropriate) can determine the utility of a particular performance. Second, she maintains that professionals are not in a position to decide which performance issues are most relevant or have the biggest impact on the person's life. Third, she explains that using professional judgment to rate performance only reinforces persons' belief that they are not active participants in the process of solving problems in their own lives. To resolve these issues in evaluation, Pollock (1993) and others (e.g., Pollock, Baptiste, Law, McColl, Opzoomer, & Polatajko, 1990; Law, Baptiste, Carswell-Opzoomer, McColl, Polatajko, & Pollock, 1991) suggest that we embrace a person-centered approach to evaluation.

The idea of person-centered care has grown out of a shift in social policies. In previous decades, persons with various disabilities have been viewed as outcasts, burdens to society, punishment for family transgressions, recipients of our benevolence, or the responsibility of a socially conscious government and society. The Kennedy era in the United States saw the beginning of the recognition of the potential of persons with disabilities to contribute to family and community life. From this initial change, many developments in social policy have caused a shift toward more and more positive views toward persons with disabilities. We now have federal laws and regulations that compel us to include persons with disabilities in schools, workplaces, and community facilities.

Having a person-centered focus in evaluation means that professionals understand and value the importance of a person's (and the family's) perspectives about life goals and priorities. In a person-centered approach, the professional frames the evaluation process with knowledge about the person's needs and desires. Even though providers in various professions have developed expertise in a wide range of areas, a person-centered approach requires that the provider only evaluate aspects of performance that are related to the person's and family's expressed needs and desires. For occupational therapists, this means that the contexts and the person's skills and performance areas must be related to the performance problems that the person and family have identified. For example, if a couple wishes for the wife to care for her husband by providing the primary support for his dressing activities, then the occupational therapist's responsibility is to evaluate what will be necessary to support the partners in this goal. In a person-centered approach, it would be inappropriate to evaluate the husband's skills for dressing himself. Rather, the occupational therapist would focus on the husband's current status for participating, the wife's skills to provide dressing cues and supports safely, and the contextual supports and adaptations that might be necessary for successful dressing, both in the hospital and at home.

Sometimes it is hard for professionals who have invested a great deal of energy in developing their expertise to turn away from what they perceive as control over the therapeutic situation. In a person-centered approach to evaluation and services, professionals recognize that their expertise is *best* applied within the needs of persons' lives. Meeting the criterion of relevance in the person's life also carries with it the opportunity for incidental learning; the person and family can begin to understand what a profession *really* has to offer when they can see it affect the satisfaction they feel with their own lives. Additionally, a person-centered approach affords professionals the opportunity to apply their discipline's expertise in the *most* creative ways. The purpose of occupational therapy is never more apparent than when performance is facilitated and a person's life becomes more satisfying.

The Canadian Occupational Performance Measure (COPM): A Model for Person-Centered Evaluation

In 1987, Law and colleagues, as part of a decade-long Canadian quality assurance project (see *Toward outcome measures in occupational therapy* H39-114/1987E), established 10 criteria for a quality occupational performance outcome measure:

1. It is based on the Model of Occupational Performance.
2. It is focused on performance in self-care, productivity, and leisure as the primary outcome.

3. It considers performance components (physical, mental-emotional, sociocultural and spiritual) as secondary outcomes, measured only for their contribution to occupational performance.
4. It considers the client's environment, developmental stage, life roles, and motivation.
5. It is sensitive to clinical change relevant to occupational therapy goals including development, restoration and maintenance of function, and prevention of disability.
6. It is not diagnosis-specific.
7. It is modular for use in whole or in part.
8. It incorporates measurement properties of reliability, responsiveness, and validity.
9. It is usable in terms of format, administration, time, ease of scoring, and client acceptability.
10. It can be scored numerically (Law et. al., 1991, pp. 6–7).

The group members originally set out to find outcome measure(s) that met these criteria, so they could inform their colleagues about this method of evaluation. They identified 136 measures originally, but only 54 measures met the first and second criteria; the others only addressed the third criterion, i.e., evaluation of performance components (n = 82). None of the rest of the measures met all the criteria the group had established; some were unpublished, others did not address roles, environment, or performance as the occupational performance model would suggest. This led the group to develop a new measure that would meet all of the criteria and that contained some of the more clever evaluation methods from those reviewed (Law et. al., 1991).

The COPM is designed to be administered in a semistructured interview and incorporates a five-step process: problem definition, problem weighting, scoring, reassessment, and follow-up. During problem definition, the therapist explores with the person and family whether they are having any difficulties with performance in daily life; the therapist gives examples of daily life activities in self-care, productivity, and leisure to assist the interviewee(s) in thinking about possible performance issues. The emphasis in this step is to find out what the person *needs, wants,* or *is expected* to perform as part of daily life. For any areas for which the person expresses the need or desire, the therapist determines whether the person is satisfied with current performance. Whenever the person expresses inability or dissatisfaction with performance, the therapist probes to discover what might be creating the barrier to performance.

Second, the therapist and person served must "weight the problems." The person weights each problem listed on a 1–10 scale (1 = not important, 10 = extremely important). Then the person selects up to five problems as most critical and rates her or his own performance and satisfaction with current performance. For scoring, the therapist multiplies importance with performance and importance with satisfaction to obtain weighted performance and satisfaction scores.

Reassessment and follow-up occur after intervention has proceeded as part of comprehensive service provision. In studies thus far, the COPM has been shown to have the capacity to document changes in performance and satisfaction across ages and types of disabilities (Pollock, 1993).

Best practice in occupational therapy evaluation necessitates embracing a person-centered approach to evaluation now and in the future. It is no longer acceptable to impose ideas upon persons who have performance needs and their families. We must join with persons and families to discover the best use of our occupational therapy knowledge and expertise on their behalf. Person-centered approaches afford us the opportunity to be relevant to persons' lives as they live them.

Conducting Contextually Relevant Evaluations

Persons perform daily life tasks in particular contexts. Even if an occupational therapist evaluates a person in a medical center clinic, this is a context that will have some influence on the person's performance. Perhaps all the unfamiliar equipment and supplies will be distracting. The therapist's expectation of performance might make the person anxious. Without prior knowledge about the person's lifestyle, the therapist might set up the evaluation context in a way that is confusing to the person. The therapist's kind and engaging affect also might facilitate performance in areas in which the person more typically performs poorly, due to lack of interest. We cannot consider the meaning of performance during any evaluation without considering the context in which the performance occurred. In order for occupational therapists to be systematic in considering context, Dunn, Brown, & McGuigan (1994) created a framework for thinking about performance in context.

A FRAMEWORK FOR CONSIDERING PERFORMANCE IN CONTEXT

Dunn, Brown, & McGuigan (1994) proposed a framework for considering performance in context, the *Ecology of Human Performance* (EHP). There are four assumptions underlying this framework:

- persons and their contexts are unique and dynamic
- contrived contexts are different than natural contexts
- occupational therapy practice involves promoting self-determination and inclusion of persons with disabilities in all aspects of society
- independence means meeting your wants and needs (Dunn, McClain, Brown, & Youngstrom, in press).

Underlying Assumptions of the Ecology of Human Performance

Persons and their contexts are unique and dynamic. We cannot understand a person we are evaluating without understanding the person's context. In the EHP framework, context includes not only the physical characteristics of the environment, but also the social, cultural, and temporal features of the environment (Dunn, Brown, & McGuigan, 1994; AOTA, 1994). Even in the context of the same family, siblings experience their world differently and develop different interests and skills. We must consider the unique nature of each person and how contexts influence that person's experiences. These transactions form the basis of the meaning that persons derive from their life experiences.

There is a dynamic relationship between persons and their contexts. The context can change based on what persons do, and changes in the context can affect how persons react as well. We set up our personal hygiene products and materials to facilitate our own rituals. Our performance changes when the arrangement of these products and materials is different (for example, when in a hotel room). Persons have a range of performance abilities based on the transaction between themselves and their contexts. During the evaluation process, we are attempting to determine the person's performance range, not just the person's skills and difficulties. Although we must know what the person's skills and difficulties are, this knowledge is inadequate without knowing what the person is interested in and where the person is likely to be conducting various aspects of daily life.

Contrived contexts are different than natural contexts. Because of the service systems within which occupational therapists work, it is often the case that evaluations occur in contexts designed for specialized services (e.g., clinical settings or acute-care settings). When we conduct evaluations in these specialized settings, we also must consider the possible differences in performance in more natural settings, such as the workplace or home. Sometimes performance will be better than typical performance in contrived settings, because contrived settings control some features of the context that might be disruptive to the person. This control enables us to see optimal performance, but we must consider therapeutic interventions based on typical performance needs, not optimal ones. Otherwise, we might conclude incorrectly that the person is unable to perform when we evaluate in contrived contexts, whereas the familiarity of a natural context might support better performance. We must be vigilant about finding out as much as we can about performance in natural settings, because these are the settings that matter to the person's life.

Occupational therapy practice involves promoting self-determination and inclusion of persons with disabilities in all aspects of society. The overall goal of occupational therapy services is to support persons in living a satisfying life. We must be sure to find out what persons and their families prioritize as part of our comprehensive evaluation processes. Additionally, as occupational therapy personnel, we must advocate for persons who have performance needs, so that they have access to all the community environments that will enable them to live satisfying lives. We must consider it part of our professional responsibility to ensure that the persons we serve and their families can participate in all the community activities that will contribute to the satisfaction of their lives. This might mean that part of our evaluation and services will include visiting the workplace to identify possible adaptations, or speaking to peers and supervisors about routines of the day that support or create barriers to performance. Occupational therapists' responsibility to the persons we serve extends into the daily contexts that affect their lives.

Independence means meeting your wants and needs. The American Occupational Therapy Association (AOTA) has an official position on the meaning of *independence* (AOTA, 1996). Independence occurs when persons are able to manage their lives to obtain what they want and need. Traditionally, independence has meant that persons actually *performed* the tasks. In our profession, however, we have taken a stand that persons might make decisions about how they want to use their resources, and this might include employing someone else to do a needed task (e.g., taking clothing to a laundromat), making an adaptation in the environment to make the task easier (e.g., using a step stool to reach cabinets), or soliciting help from family, coworkers, or friends. The important part of independence is a person's ability to know what needs to be done and finding a way to get it done; it is not necessary to do the task one's self to be considered independent.

Although this is obvious for persons without disabilities, we sometimes forget this broad view of independence when persons have disabilities. When evaluating persons who have performance needs, adaptations of the task or context to support performance must be explored as part of comprehensive evaluation. All of us use adaptations to support our daily life (e.g., using Post-it® notes, jar openers, long-handled barbeque tools). Identifying ways to support one's own independent performance must not be considered a negative feature. When persons have disabilities, there is a temptation to immediately consider these supports as indications that the person has a problem. The more progressive view is that sometimes the context needs to be adjusted to be more "user friendly" for those who perform in that context. This is not a reflection on the person's skills and abilities but rather an acknowledgement that sometimes contexts contain barriers to optimal performance for certain people.

Core Concepts of the Ecology of Human Performance Framework

The EHP framework includes person, context, and performance variables, and the transactions among them. Figure 4.1 illustrates the relationships

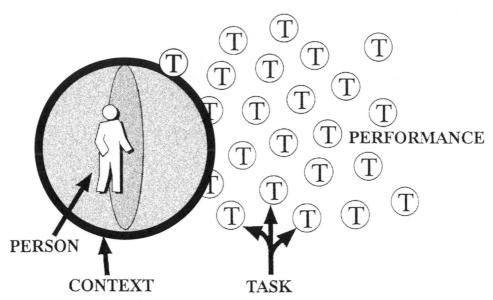

PERFORMANCE

PERSON

CONTEXT   **TASK**

Figure 4.1. Schemata for the *Ecology of Human Performance* framework. Persons are imbedded in their contexts. An infinite variety of tasks exists around every person. Performance occurs as a result of the person interacting with context to engage in tasks.

Dunn, W., Brown, C., & McGuigan, A. (1994). The ecology of human performance: A framework for considering the effect of context. *American Journal of Occupational Therapy, 48(7),* 595–607. Reprinted with permission.

among these variables. The person is imbedded in the context, just as the Tootsie Roll® center is imbedded in a Tootsie Roll Pop®. You cannot see the person ("the Tootsie Roll®") without looking through the context ("the candy coating"). Tasks are represented by the circles with the Ts in them; they surround the person in context. According to the EHP framework, tasks are independent of persons and contexts. Theoretically, all tasks are available to everyone; it is the person's skills, interests, and the features of a particular context that determine which tasks are within that person's performance range (the shaded section to the right of the diagram). In this figure, the context serves as a "lens" that transacts with the person's skills to project onto the universe of tasks that are available.

Persons can have limited skills, abilities, and experience due to a variety of factors (for example, developmental disability, head trauma, mental illness). With limited "person" skills, the transactions between the person and the context are more limited. The person is less able to take advantage of supporting features of the context. A child with attentional deficits has the same context as other children in the classroom, but may not be able to take advantage of the cues in this context that guide appropriate behavior. For example, the other children might quickly notice the teacher's cues to quiet down after recess, but the child with attentional difficulties may not understand these cues, thereby increasing the chances for inappropriate behavior. When the

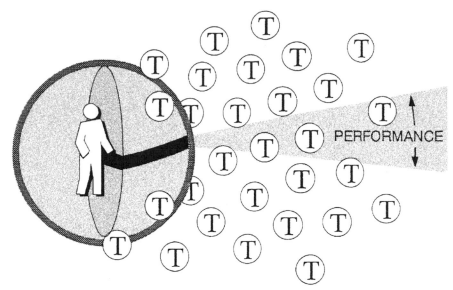

Figure 4.2. Schemata of a person with limited skills and abilities within the *Ecology of Human Performance* framework. Although context is still useful, the person has fewer skills and abilities to "look through" context and derive meaning. This limits the person's performance range.

Dunn, W., Brown, C., & McGuigan, A. (1994). The ecology of human performance: A framework for considering the effect of context. *American Journal of Occupational Therapy, 48(7),* 595–607. Reprinted with permission.

person has more limited skills, the transaction between the person and context creates a more limited performance range; Figure 4.2 depicts this transaction.

It is also possible for the context to be limited. We have all experienced limited contexts in which we have attempted to do something without adequate equipment, supplies, help from others, or time. When the context is limited, this will also affect the performance range (see Figure 4.3). Even when persons have good skills and abilities and the context is limited, the transaction between the person and context will lead to a limited performance range. An expert skier who lives on the plains of the Midwest will not be able to demonstrate those skills without traveling to a new context.

Sometimes people who have disabilities also live and work in limited contexts. This compounds the problem of performance, because both person and context variables are diminished. The performance range can be very restricted in this situation. Occupational therapists must attend to both of these parts of the transaction in comprehensive evaluation to ensure that all factors related to the performance range are considered.

Applying the Ecology of Human Performance Framework to Comprehensive Evaluation

If occupational therapists employ the EHP framework to design their comprehensive and ongoing evaluation plans, three factors must be addressed. Occupa-

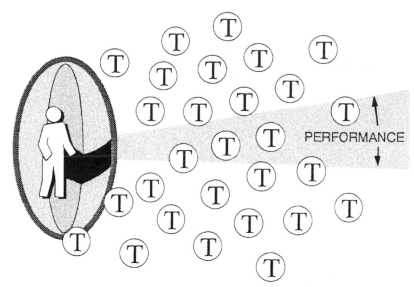

Figure 4.3. Schemata of a limited context within the *Ecology of Human Performance* framework. The person has adequate skills and abilities, but the context does not provide resources needed to perform. In this situation, performance range is limited.

Dunn, W., Brown, C., & McGuigan, A. (1994). The ecology of human performance: A framework for considering the effect of context. *American Journal of Occupational Therapy, 48(7),* 595–607. Reprinted with permission.

tional therapists are concerned with performance in daily life; therefore, the most important aspect of any occupational therapy evaluation is performance. In the EHP framework, performance has two features: consideration of what the person wants and needs to do, and assessment of actual performance. To determine what the person wants and needs to do, we talk to the person, the family, friends, other care providers, and significant players in the person's life (e.g., a coworker, boss, minister, neighbors). Our objective is to determine what matters in the person's life. To determine actual performance, occupational therapists can conduct interviews about how performance looks in the natural contexts and how satisfying that performance is for the person. We also observe the person's performance of tasks, either through informal evaluation or with formal assessments of daily life. Dunn, Brown, McClain, & Westman (1994) provided a series of worksheets for summarizing evaluation data using an EHP framework. Table 4.1 is a summary of a Task Analysis worksheet, which is a simplified version of an ecological inventory. On this table, the professional describes typical performance of the task and the performance of the person being evaluated. Table 4.2 contains a completed Task Analysis worksheet on Ellie, a young woman who wishes to cook in her apartment. We see that Ellie has some supports to cooking successfully. Other chapters in this text cover evaluation of task performance in more detail than is possible here.

■ *Table 4.1.* Task Analysis Worksheet

Name: Task:

Typical Performance of Task	This Person's Performance of Task

Dunn, W., Brown, C., McClain, L., & Westman, K. (1994). The ecology of human performance: A contextual perspective on human occupation. In C.B. Royeen (Ed.), *AOTA self study series: The practice of the future: Putting occupation back into therapy* (Chapter I). Bethesda, MD: American Occupational Therapy Association. Reprinted with permission.

■ *Table 4.2.* Summary of Task Analysis Worksheet

Name: Ellie   Task: Menu preparation

Typical Performance of Task	This Person's Performance of Task
This task requires background skills such as sustained attention, visual motor skills, and memory.	Community-living coach has limited the menu preparation to dinner menu planning only.
Provides changing visual stimuli (paper to book as she records).	Coach provides verbal cues to prompt Ellie to get all parts completed and to include variety.
Requires problem solving and generalization of learning (e.g., how to obtain variety, how to organize the task).	Cookbook has tabs on sections so Ellie can find them easily and to cue her that there are other sections to consider.
Provides visual cues (e.g., pictures in cookbook).	Coach provides paper with weekly schedule already marked on it.

Dunn, W., Brown, C., McClain, L., & Westman, K. (1994). The ecology of human performance: A contextual perspective on human occupation. In C.B. Royeen (Ed.), *AOTA self study series: The practice of the future: Putting occupation back into therapy* (Chapter I). Bethesda, MD: American Occupational Therapy Association. Reprinted with permission.

The second factor in comprehensive evaluation is consideration of the person's skills, abilities, and experiences. For this aspect of evaluation, occupational therapists examine sensorimotor, cognitive, and psychosocial features of the person's performance. Our purpose in evaluating these component skills is to determine what person variables might be contributing to or creating barriers to desired performance. There are many formal and informal methods of evaluating performance components; other chapters in this text address the specifics of these aspects of comprehensive evaluation. Table 4.3 contains a Data Summary worksheet to delineate the sensorimotor, cognitive, and

■ *Table 4.3.* Data Summary Worksheet

Name: Tasks:

Person Variables	Activities of Daily Living	Work/Productive Activity	Play/Leisure Performance
sensorimotor			
cognitive			
psychosocial			

Dunn, W., Brown, C., McClain, L., & Westman, K. (1994). The ecology of human performance: A contextual perspective on human occupation. In C.B. Royeen (Ed.), *AOTA self study series: The practice of the future: Putting occupation back into therapy* (Chapter I). Bethesda, MD: American Occupational Therapy Association. Reprinted with permission.

psychosocial aspects (rows) of the daily life tasks (columns) that are of interest to the person, and Table 4.4 contains a Data Summary worksheet on Ellie (Dunn et. al., 1994).

Finally, the EHP framework compels us to consider the context of performance. We must evaluate the context in order to determine possible barriers and supports in the context. The transaction between these contextual variables and the person's performance is what determines the meaning the person derives from his or her own experiences.

CONTEXTUAL EVALUATION

In spite of the fact that occupational therapy literature has always stated that environments were important, context is evaluated far less than person and performance variables. When evaluating context, there are three areas to consider. First, we must consider the physical, social, cultural, and temporal features of the contexts. Second, we must identify the possible supports and barriers to performance. Third, we must hypothesize about the meaning of performance in this context for the person being evaluated.

Letts, Law, Rigby, Cooper, Stewart, and Strong (1994) compiled a comprehensive list of assessments that help professionals record various aspects of context. Table 4.5 contains a reprinted version of the data they compiled describing 41 environmental assessments. This summary includes the name of the instrument, environmental attributes measured, environment for application, purpose, clinical utility, instrument development, and psychometric properties. These measures were largely designed by those in other professions than occupational therapy, suggesting that this is a salient issue for others as well.

■ *Table 4.4.* Data Summary Worksheet for Ellie

Name: Ellie   Tasks: (this worksheet for menu preparation only)

Person Variables	Activities of Daily Living	Work/Productive Activity	Play/Leisure Performance
sensorimotor		Flips through the cookbook easily. Scans and finds recipes quickly. Continues to work on task with TV on.	
cognitive		Remembers recipes she's eaten before and talks about them. Once identifying a section, tends to remain in that section for several selections. Recognizes need for main dish and dessert, but forgets about the need for side dishes. Stays on task throughout time. Has difficulty deciding if all food groups have been included.	
psychosocial		Attached to this cookbook; it is just like her mother's; reluctant to move to recipe cards.	

Dunn, W., Brown, C., McClain, L., & Westman, K. (1994). The ecology of human performance: A contextual perspective on human occupation. In C.B. Royeen (Ed.), *AOTA self study series: The practice of the future: Putting occupation back into therapy* (Chapter I). Bethesda, MD: American Occupational Therapy Association. Reprinted with permission.

Physical, social, cultural, and temporal features of context. Occupational therapists use skilled observations and interviews to determine the physical, social, cultural, and temporal features of relevant contexts. The physical features of context include the objects, terrain, layout, and structures of the environment. Social features include the persons, interaction styles, and relationships within the context. Culture in a context includes the expectations of stakeholders, such as family, community, ethnic groups, or coworkers. Temporal features of context refer to expectations related to age, calendar time, or stage of disability. Table 4.6 contains a format for summarizing contextual data; Table 4.7 contains data about Ellie (Dunn et. al., 1994).

A common way to evaluate the features of context is through ecological assessment. Here we observe the natural course of activities in a particular context, and record our observations. This usually includes documenting what typical persons in this context do to engage in and complete necessary tasks, what the person of interest does to complete the tasks, and possible ways to bridge the gap between the two. Figure 4.4 contains an example of an ecological assessment for a young child in a preschool program; teachers and parents want her to learn to eat her snack with the other children. (See Table 4.2 for another example of an ecological inventory.)

■ *Table 4.5.* Environmental Assessments

Instrument Title and Author	Environmental Attributes Measured	Environmental Application	Purpose— to Determine	Clinical Utility	Instrument Development	Psychometric Testing
1. The Accessibility Checklist (Goltsman et al., 1992)	Physical	Community	Accessibility of buildings and outdoor facilities	Survey checklists for a large number of physical spaces (e.g. playgrounds, retail areas) Useful in consultation with other professionals	Manual with clear instructions Based on ADA, UFAS, California Building Code	Content validity during scale construction No reliability testing
2. Assessment of Home Environments (Yarrow et al., 1975)	Social and cultural	Family	Adequacy of the infant's early developmental environment at home (ages: newborn to 6 months)	Structured observations Limited instructions Useful for early intervention	Nominal data Content not justified No manual	One interrater reliability study No validity testing
3. Assessment Tool (Maltais et al., 1989)	Physical	Individual	Environmental barriers in a house, specific to functional limitations of an elderly person	Structured questionnaire Clear instructions Useful to promote independence of clients in their homes	Manual available Nominal data Norms available	One interrater reliability study One content validity study
4. Behavioral Environment Assessment Technique (Whitehead et al., 1984)	Social	Community	How adults behave in or use institutional space	Structured observations Useful for institutional planning, evaluation of environmental modifications	No manual	One reliability study One content validity study using factor analysis
5. Child Care Centre Accessibility Checklist (Metro Toronto Community Services, 1991)	Physical	Community	Barrier-free accessibility of child care centers	Direct observation and measurement of the environment Clear instructions Useful for determining physical accessibility	Manual available Nominal data Norms: based on ANSI standards and Ontario building code	Reliability unknown Content validity determined based on instrument development

6. Classroom Environment Scale (Trickett & Moos, 1973)	Social	Individual Community	Aspects of classroom psychosocial environment salient to students and teachers	Questionnaire 3 forms, 90 items for each Useful for consultation within a classroom	Manual, with clear instructions Items selected based on theory and expert opinion Nominal data Norms available	One reliability study: internal consistency Content validity tested using factor analysis
7. Classroom Environment Index (Stern & Walker, 1971)	Social Cultural	Individual Community	Student's perception of the classroom environment	Self-administered questionnaire 300 true/false statements Useful to describe classroom variables (e.g., achievement level) and student-environment fit	Manual available Item selection based on experts, literature, and testing in schools Norms available Nominal data	Internal consistency tested Factor analysis and discriminative validity tested
8. Disability Rights Guide (Goldman, 1991)	Economic and Institutional	Individual Community	Problems affecting persons with disabilities in accessing their community	Self-report questionnaires address institutional barriers to accessibility Useful for community planning, advocacy	Questionnaires are contained within textbook Content based on ADA Nominal data	Unknown reliability Content validity based on instrument development
9. Environment Assessment Index (Poresky, 1987)	Physical Social	Family	Educational and developmental quality of the home environment for children ages 3 to 11 years living in rural communities	Questionnaire; structured interview and observations Clear instructions Useful for direct service, family education, program evaluation	Manual available from author Item selection based on literature review and expert opinion Nominal data	One reliability study: internal consistency Validity: content validity with factor analysis; concurrent and predictive correlations
10. Environment Assessment Scale (Kannegieter, 1986)	Economic and Institutional	Individual	Characteristics of the occupational therapy clinical environment as perceived by the psychiatric client	Structured interview Useful for individual program planning, program evaluation	Manual available from unpublished source No norms Nominal data Comprehensive item selection	Internal consistency and test–retest reliability established Criterion and content validity testing underway

continued

■ *Table 4.5.* continued

Instrument Title and Author	Environmental Attributes Measured	Environmental Application	Purpose— to Determine	Clinical Utility	Instrument Development	Psychometric Testing
11. Environmental Competence Questionnaire (CMHC, 1982)	Physical Social	Individual Community	Competence of elderly persons living independently in their homes	Questionnaire; structured interview Instructions not provided Useful for direct service to adults with physical limitations	No manual Item selection appears adequate Nominal data	Unknown reliability and validity
12. Environmental Grid Description Assessment (Dunning, 1972)	Physical Social Cultural	Individual Family	Person's relationship with environmental space, persons, and tasks	Semi-structured interview No instructions Useful as a client-centered assessment of occupational choice	No manual Item selection appears adequate	Unknown reliability and validity
13. Environment Preference Questionnaire (Kaplan, 1977)	Physical	Individual Community	Individual differences in environmental preferences	Questionnaire, respondent can complete independently Clear instructions Useful in direct service	Manual available from author Item selection based on literature review, expert opinion Ordinal data	Reliability; internal consistency Content validity based on factor analysis
14. Environmental Response Inventory (McKechnie, 1974)	Social	Individual Family Community	Differences in the ways persons habitually interact with the environment	Questionnaire, can be completed independently Clear instructions Useful for career, life-style counseling, program planning	Manual available Item selection based on literature review, limited by factor analysis Ordinal data	Reliability unknown Content, construct, criterion validity established

15. Functional Requirements in the Physical Environment (United Nations, 1981)	Physical Economic and Institutional	Community Province and Country	Features of the built environment for accessibility by persons with physical, sensory, or cognitive disability	Checklist Clear instructions Useful for community consultation about accessibility	Manual available from United Nations Item selection comprehensive Nominal data	Unknown reliability Content validity based on instrument development
16. Home Observation for Measurement of the Environment (Caldwell & Bradley, 1979)	Physical Social Cultural	Family	Adequacy of a child's early developmental environment at home (ages: newborn to 6 years)	Structured observations and interview with parents Clear instructions Useful for consultation and family education	Manual available Item selection based on factor analysis Nominal data	Internal consistency and test–retest reliability tested, adequate statistical results Content and construct validity established
17. Home Modification Workbook (Adaptive Environments Center, 1988)	Physical	Individual	Home safety and potential for independent function of elderly individuals' homes	Questionnaire and observations in checklist format Useful to structure modifications to home for an individual's needs	Manual available Content justified Nominal data	Unknown reliability Content validity addressed during instrument development
18. Importance, Locus, and Range of Activities Checklist (Hulicka et al., 1975)	Physical Social Cultural	Individual	Individual's perceived latitude of choice in ADL	Interview with checklist Clear instructions Useful for client-centered program planning	No manual available Item selection process not well described Ordinal data	Test–retest reliability established Construct and content validity tested
19. Infant-Toddler Environment Rating Scale (Harms et al., 1990)	Social	Community	Quality of center-based child care for children up to 30 months of age	Structured observation Clear instructions Useful for consultation, program planning	Manual available Item selection based on other scales Ordinal data	Interrater, test–retest and internal consistency established Content and criterion validity established

continued

■ *Table 4.5.* continued

Instrument Title and Author	Environmental Attributes Measured	Environmental Application	Purpose— to Determine	Clinical Utility	Instrument Development	Psychometric Testing
20. Interpersonal Support Evaluation List (Cohen et al., 1985)	Social	Individual	Availability of social support for adults	Self-report questionnaire Clear, concise instructions Useful for direct service, consultation	Manual available from author Item selection comprehensive Nominal data	Internal consistency and test–retest reliability established Concurrent and construct validity established
21. Life Stressors and Social Resources Inventory (Moos, Fenn, & Billings, 1988)	Physical Social Cultural	Individual Family Community	Common life stressors and social resources that influence well-being	Semi-structured interview Clear instructions Useful for direct service, consultation and community planning	Manual available Item selection based on literature review and expert opinion Nominal data	Internal consistency established Content validity based on factor analysis
22. Modification Checklist (CMHC, 1988)	Physical	Individual Community	Accessibility barriers of a house or apartment	Checklist based on observations Clear instructions Useful for direct service	Manual available Item selection based on opinions of clinical experts, disabled persons, rehabilitation centers, architects, etc. Nominal data	Unknown reliability Content validity based on instrument development
23. Multilevel Assessment Instrument (Lawton et al., 1982)	Social	Individual	Well-being and behavioral competence of elderly persons at home and in community	Structured interview Limited instructions Useful for comprehensive assessment of function in an environment	No manual Item selection based on literature review and expert opinion Nominal data	Internal consistency established Content validity established

24. Multiphasic Environmental Assessment Procedure (Moos & Lemke, 1988)	Physical Economic Institutional Social	Community	Adequacy of sheltered care settings	Structured questionnaire in five parts Clear instructions Useful for consultation in sheltered care settings	Manual available Item selection based on theory, literature review, and experts Ordinal and interval data Norms available	Internal consistency, interrater and test–retest reliability established Content, construct validity established
25. Need Satisfaction of Activity Interview (Tickle & Yerxa, 1981)	Social	Individual	Person's preferences for activities within his/her environment	Interview Clear instructions Useful for direct service, program planning	No manual Instructions available in published paper Item selection comprehensive Descriptive data	One test–retest reliability study Content validity based on factor analysis
26. Perceived Environment Constraint Index (Wolk & Telleen, 1976)	Economic Institutional	Individual Community	Level of personal autonomy allowed in a geriatric residential setting	Self-report questionnaire Clear instructions Useful for institutional planning	Instructions available in text Item selection comprehensive Ordinal data	Unknown reliability Content validity established
27. Person-Environment Fit (Kahana, 1974)	Physical Social Cultural Economic Institutional	Individual Community	Congruence between residential environment and elderly individual	Self-report questionnaire Limited instructions Useful for long-term care planning, consultation	No manual Item selection comprehensive Nominal data	Unknown reliability and validity
28. Person-Environment Fit Scale (Coulton, 1979)	Physical Social Cultural Economic Institutional	Individual Community	Person-environment fit	Self-report questionnaire Clear instructions Useful for direct service, community consultation, and planning	Manual available from author Item selection based on literature review and expert opinion Ordinal data	Internal consistency established Content and construct validity established

continued

■ *Table 4.5.* continued

Instrument Title and Author	Environmental Attributes Measured	Environmental Application	Purpose— to Determine	Clinical Utility	Instrument Development	Psychometric Testing
29. Planner's Guide to Barrier-Free Meetings (Russell, 1980)	Physical	Community	Barrier-free accessibility of facilities for group meetings	Checklist Clear instructions Useful for consultation about accessibility	Manual available Item selection based on ANSI standards Nominal data	Unknown reliability Content validity addressed in instrument development
30. Planning Barrier-Free Libraries (National Library Service, 1981)	Physical Economic Institutional	Community	Barrier-free accessibility of public libraries	Checklist Clear instructions Useful for community consultation	Manual available Item selection based on ANSI standards, expert and consumer opinions Nominal data	Unknown reliability Content validity addressed in instrument development
31. Play History (Takata, 1969; Behnke & Fetkovich, 1984)	Physical Social Cultural	Individual Family	Child's past and present play experiences and environmental opportunities	Semi-structured interview Clear instructions Useful for direct service	No manual—instructions available from authors Item selection based on literature review Ordinal data	Interrater and test–retest reliability established Content and concurrent validity tested
32. Quality of Life Interview (Lehman, 1988)	Social	Individual	Satisfaction in nine life domains	Interview Clear instructions Useful in direct, client-centered service	Manual available Item selection based on literature review Ordinal data	Internal consistency, and test–retest reliability tested Construct validity established
33. Readily Achievable Checklist (Cronburg et al., 1991)	Physical	Community	Barriers to accessibility	Structured observations and measurements Useful for obtaining public accessibility	Manual available Instructions and guidelines comprehensive	Unknown reliability Content validity addressed during instrument development

34. Safety Assessment of Function and the Environment for Rehabilitation (COTA, 1991)	Physical Social	Individual	Ability of the elderly person to function safely in his or her home	Checklist using observations and interview Clear instructions Useful for community-based practice, discharge planning	Manual available from author Item selection based on literature review, clinician and consumer opinion Nominal data	Internal consistency established Content and construct validity tested
35. School—Quick Checklist (Ontario Ministry of Education, 1986)	Physical	Community	Accessibility barriers of schools Modification requirements	Checklist; observations Clear instructions Useful for school consultations	Manual available Item selection based on building code standards Nominal data	Unknown reliability Content validity addressed in instrument development
36. Source Book (Kelly & Snell, 1989)	Physical	Individual	Environmental barriers in a house, specific to functional limitations of a person with physical disabilities	Structured questionnaire, observations, and guidelines Clear instructions Useful for direct service, consultation	Manual available Item selection based on literature review and expert opinion Nominal data Standards based on ANSI and CSA	No reliability testing Content validity addressed in instrument development
37. Tenant Interview (Howell, 1980)	Social	Community	Behavioral preferences of adults living in congregate housing	Structured interview Clear instructions Useful for program planning	Manual available Item selection based on literature review and expert opinion Nominal data	Unknown reliability and validity
38. Therapeutic Environment Guidelines (Chambers et al., 1988)	Economic Institutional	Community	Attributes of residential lodges for adults needing long-term care	Checklist to use with observations and unstructured interview Clear instructions Useful for consultation	No manual available Item selection based on literature review and expert opinions Ordinal data	Unknown reliability Content validity based on instrument development

continued

■ *Table 4.5.* continued

Instrument Title and Author	Environmental Attributes Measured	Environmental Application	Purpose—to Determine	Clinical Utility	Instrument Development	Psychometric Testing
39. UCP–OT Initial Evaluation (Colvin & Korn, 1984)	Physical	Family	Physical barriers to the care of children with cerebral palsy within their own home environment	Semi-structured questionnaire using observations and interview Clear instructions Useful in community practice	No manual available Item selection based on ANSI standards Nominal data	Unknown reliability Content validity addressed in instrument development
40. Work Environment Scale (Moos, 1981)	Social	Individual Community	Interpersonal environment of workplace as perceived by employers and staff members	Structured questionnaire Clear instructions Useful for direct service, workplace consultations	Manual available Item selection based on theory, literature review, expert opinion Nominal data	Internal consistency and test–retest reliability established Content validity based on factor analysis
41. Workplace Workbook (Mueller, 1990)	Physical	Individual	Environmental barriers in a workplace	Structured observations and measurements for barrier-free accessibility Useful for preparing the work environment for a person with a physical disability	Manual available Content justified Nominal data	Unknown reliability Content validity addressed during instrument development

Note: ADA = American With Disabilities Act, UFAS = Uniform Federal Accessibility Standards, ANSI = American National Standards Institute, ADL = activities of daily living, CMHC = Canada Mortgage and Housing Corporation, COTA = Community Occupational Therapists and Associates, UCP–OT = United Cerebral Palsy–Occupational Therapy, CSA = Canadian Standards Association.

■ *Table 4.6.* **Context Data Worksheet**

Name:

	Code*
Physical	
Social	
Cultural	
Temporal	
*Code: s = supporting factor; b = barrier to performance; ? = could be either	

Dunn, W., Brown, C., McClain, L., & Westman, K. (1994). The ecology of human performance: A contextual perspective on human occupation. In C.B. Royeen (Ed.), *AOTA self study series: The practice of the future: Putting occupation back into therapy* (Chapter I). Bethesda, MD: American Occupational Therapy Association. Reprinted with permission.

■ *Table 4.7.* **Context Data Worksheet**

Name: Ellie

	Code*
Physical	
Ellie lives in a community apartment	s
The apartment has open living areas—living room open with kitchen.	?
The kitchen is a U-shaped design.	?
Social	
Ellie works in a day-care center.	s
She does laundry with a neighbor.	s
She goes out with friends each week.	s
She visits family once a week.	s
Cultural	
Ellie receives support from a community living program.	s
She lives in an apartment with others she has known through school.	s
She lives in the city, with close access to community resources like grocery stores, drug stores; workers know Ellie and enjoy helping her in their places of business.	s
Temporal	
As a young adult, Ellie wants to live in her own place.	s
She enjoys her independence from her family and the group home from which she moved.	s
Her coach expresses concern about her skills related to expectations.	s
*Code: s = supporting factor; b = barrier to performance; ? = could be either	

Dunn, W., Brown, C., McClain, L., & Westman, K. (1994). The ecology of human performance: A contextual perspective on human occupation. In C.B. Royeen (Ed.), *AOTA self study series: The practice of the future: Putting occupation back into therapy* (Chapter I). Bethesda, MD: American Occupational Therapy Association. Reprinted with permission.

Figure 4.4. Ecologically Based Individualized Adaptation Inventory

Environment: Classroom snack time area   **Activity:** Eating snack, drinking juice

A Nonhandi-capped Toddler Inventory Plan	An Inventory of Beth	Skills Beth Can Probably Acquire	Skills Beth May Not Acquire	Adaptation Possibilities	Observation	
					Assessment	Daily Plan
Move to snack area.	Cannot get to table by self.	Can learn to walk.		Adult can assist by using facilitation.	Beth walked well when facilitation at hips was used.	Teacher will fade assistance as demonstrated by therapist. Aim for walking well with one hand held within a month.
Position self at table.	Cannot get chair out to sit down.	Can learn to get chair out; rotate to sit.		Adult can assist with pulling chair out & facilitating rotation to sit.	She pulled out chair with hand over hand; rotated & sat with facilitation from trunk.	Fade assistance in hand over hand for pulling chair; aim for pulling w/o increased tone in arms; teacher will fade facilitation for rotating to sit as demonstrated by therapist.
Take utensils when passed out.	Can grasp large items.					Beth will take utensils by self.
Take food when passed out.	Can grasp large items (cookies) but not small pieces.		May not learn to grasp very small items.	Try small toddler fork for small pieces or only give large finger foods.	Fork worked with "stabbable" foods.	Use toddler fork.
Hold cup for liquid to be poured into.	Cup is held sideways.	Can learn to hold cup straight.		Use cup with two handles.	Beth held cup sides with hands through handles.	Use two-handled cup.
Eat food.	Can finger feed.					Beth will finger feed by self.
Drink liquid.	Can drink but not hold cup to mouth.	Can learn to hold cup.		Adult assistance to facilitate cup to mouth pattern.	Minimal help was needed to raise cup to mouth.	Fade assistance to verbal cues "pick up cup" to no cues.
Request more if desired.	Vocalizes for more.		May not learn to talk.	Use picture communication board during snack.	A picture board with cup and correct food was used when prompted "Do you want more?" She vocalized at same time.	Teacher will make picture board each day to include cup and correct food. Place board in front of Beth and watch for her to use spontaneously. If she does not indicate that she wants more, verbally prompt. Use magnetic stove board and magnet pictures. Reinforce all joint points and vocalizations.

Sample ecological assessment for a preschooler at snack time. Baumgart, D., Brown, L., Pumpian, I., Nisbet, J., Ford, A., Sweet, M., Messina, R., & Schroeder, J. (1982). Principle of partial participation and individualized adaptations in educational programs for severely handicapped students. *The Journal of The Association for the Severely Handicapped, 7(2),* 17–27. Used with permission.

Contextual supports and barriers to performance. Many of the contextual measures listed in Table 4.5 offer occupational therapists methods for identifying features of various environments. The next step in comprehensive evaluation of context is to consider how the features in the environment seem to be supporting or creating barriers to performance. It is important to remember that each person reacts to contextual variables in unique ways; what might be a support to one person may be a barrier to performance for another person. For example, the TV playing during mealtime preparation may only provide background noise or entertainment for one person, but it may be so distracting for another person that the meal would be delayed. The social pressures of a peer group may compel one adolescent to behave maladaptively, but may have no impact on another young person. The fact that a professional has gathered the objective data about the context is not adequate to make decisions about performance. Professionals have to consider the impact of those contextual features on the performance of the person being evaluated.

The two primary methods for determining whether contextual variables create supports or barriers are interviewing and skilled observation. Many times, we do not know initially whether a contextual feature is a support or barrier, and we must observe longer or ask more questions to determine the correct conclusion. For example, in Table 4.7 we see that Ellie lives in an apartment with open living areas. This arrangement could be a support if she enjoys cooking for others and is supported by their company as she works. However, this open arrangement could be a barrier if she needs fewer visual and auditory distractions so she can concentrate on cooking tasks. In conversations with Ellie and her community living coach, and through observations of performance, the therapist can determine whether this feature of her apartment will facilitate, be neutral, or to reduce performance in the kitchen.

Meaning of performance in context. The most relevant aspect of contextual evaluation is determining the meaning of the performance for the person in the particular context. A person's experiences, cultural background, and socialization opportunities contribute to meaningfulness. Although skilled therapists can observe and hypothesize about the meaning of tasks for persons, we cannot presume to know the meaning for the persons we are serving and their families, without engaging in dialogue with them. When we are trying to find out what they want and need to do, we can inquire about why those tasks are important or satisfying, or why doing them in a certain way or in a certain place is significant. We can find out from family and friends how the person's lifestyle has been constructed, and the purpose and settings for work and leisure for the person. We can inquire about the presence or absence of daily routines, the role of unexpected events, and establishment of priorities. All of this information helps to inform us about what is meaningful and what meanings are important to the persons we are serving and their families. Many times performance takes on more meaning when it is conducted in relevant contexts; poor performance in a context not relevant for the person may only indicate lack of meaningfulness of the task in that context, not lack of skill for performance. Frequently, identifying meaningfulness occurs across the evaluation and intervention phases of services.

Using Person and Performance Data Within a Context

Ultimately, the only thing that matters in person-centered and contextually relevant service provision is that the person being served and the family have the opportunity to live what is a satisfying life for them. Living a satisfying life might include developing one's own skills to a functional level, but it might also mean selecting or designing contexts that can support needed and desired task performance or finding alternative ways to meet life goals. During the evaluation process, providers must frame their inquiries around the actual life the person wants to live, even when services may be provided in a center or agency (for instance, a hospital, a clinic). Since intervention planning is based on evaluation data, the provider's goal is to ensure that evaluations include data about performance in the person's actual life.

For example, it does not matter what the child's balance score is on a standardized test if balance is not interfering with daily life activities of interest to the child and family. Our interest in the technical aspects of balance is only relevant when the person and family describe lack of satisfaction about a task and when our expertise causes us to suspect that poor balance might be interfering with this task. If a child wishes to ride bikes with the neighborhood children and cannot do so, it is appropriate to suspect balance as a barrier to this desired socialization experience. In this example, we also recognize that riding bikes with friends in the neighborhood has some inherent qualities that must be considered as well. The other children probably provide great motivation for performance; they might also be distracting to the new bike rider who has competing attention between staying on the bike and engaging with the friends. The texture and the terrain of the streets will increase the need for adaptability in postural control while on the bike. Adjustments to the bike of choice might make the task more accessible. It would also be important to know the culture of bike riding in this neighborhood with this age group; perhaps there are some expectations about tricks to be performed on the bike, such that those who cannot perform these tricks are considered less desirable group members. Artful and effective occupational therapy service provision would require that the therapist know as much of this information as possible, to create the greatest possibility for a successful outcome. Evaluation of balance is irrelevant without first considering the person's desired performance and then considering contextual features that may affect performance.

Application of Person-Centered, Contextually Relevant Evaluation Concepts

Let us consider an example of a contextually relevant person-centered evaluation process in a public school, a common life context for children.

Case Example

Samuel is an 8-year-old third grader. He completed his work in the first and second grade acceptably most of the time. He has always had trouble staying in his desk chair for any length of time, formed letters poorly when writing, and displayed frustration during art classes. In the first and second grades, the teachers were able to make changes in the classroom and with tasks so that Samuel could continue in their classes. One teacher let Samuel lie on the floor to color, while another teacher broke his work into smaller parts for him. However, the demands of third grade are more complex, and Samuel is having more trouble keeping up with assignments. He is beginning to act frustrated in class, by tearing up his work when he is not satisfied, and kicking the wall or furniture when things are not working out the way he wanted them to. The teacher does not want these behaviors to escalate, nor does she want him to lose ground in learning, so she sought help from the diagnostic team (adapted from Dunn, 1990). ■

The public school program that Samuel attends has a well-established diagnostic team, which includes occupational therapists. The team has designed a form for sketching out the initial evaluation plan for children based on the referring party's concerns; the occupational therapist has followed the team's model and created an evaluation planning form as well. Table 4.8 contains a completed occupational therapy evaluation planning form for Samuel. The form prompts the therapist to consider performance variables (skilled observations), person variables (formal, informal, and criterion-referenced tests), task variables (activity analysis) and context variables (ecological assessment).

An interdisciplinary team evaluated Samuel, so it is appropriate to summarize data from all the team members. Table 4.9 contains a summary of the team's interpretation of their evaluation data related to Samuel's performance in the classroom. The team was able to combine its knowledge about Samuel, his classroom, and the tasks he needed to perform, to document a picture of his current performance status. All the summary statements are related to the performance need expressed by his teacher. This information can then be

■ *Table 4.8.* Data Collection Plan for Samuel

Procedure	+Use	Assessment Techniques
Formal tests Norm referenceed	+ + +	Bruininks-Oseretsky Test of Motor Proficiency Sensory Integration and Praxis Test Test of Visual Perception—nonmotor Test of Visual Motor Skills Motor Free Test of Visual Perception Peabody Gross and Fine Motor Scale Beery Test of Visual Motor Integration Other, specify _____
Formal tests Criterion referenced		Brigance Inventory (specify _____) Hawaii Early Learning Profile Developmental Programming for Infants and Young Children Learning Accomplishment Profile Other, specify _____
Informal tests		Gross motor checklist Fine motor checklist Other, specify _____
Skilled observations	+ + +	Clinical observations Classroom performance (specify: seatwork) Gym class Recess Lunch room Other, specify: during directed instruction
Interviews	 + + +	Student Classroom teacher Special educator Team coordinator/case manager Parents/guardians Others, specify _____
Environmental/ecological assessment	+	Classroom Playground Lunchroom Gym Bathrooms Others, specify _____
Records review	+	School records Health records Evaluation records from _____

Activity analysis
  Analyze typical task perfor-
  mance and unique features
  of this environment
	+
	+
		Task a: seatwork
		Task b: participation in group instruction
		Task c: _____

Dunn, W. (1990). Clinical case workbook I. In C.B. Royeen (Ed.), *AOTA self study series: Assessing function* (Lesson 11). Bethesda, MD: American Occupational Therapy Association. Reprinted with permission.

■ *Table 4.9.* **Interpretive Summary of Samuel's Evaluation Data**

Strengths related to how person/task/context variables are affecting performance

The teacher believes that Samuel knows answers in class in spite of the fact that he has done poorly on homework.

Prior classroom adaptations have helped Samuel.

Samuel participates in class activities and discussions and seems capable of following group instruction.

Samuel has friends in the class and in his neighborhood at home.

When Samuel completes assignments, his writing is readable.

Samuel works at his desk for approximately 7–11 minutes.

Samuel works with the typical movement, sound, and activity in the classroom.

Samuel's desk is the proper size to support his work patterns.

Samuel enjoys putting puzzles together with family and friends; he tends to look for pieces, but engages others to place the pieces into the puzzle.

Concerns related to how person/task/context variables are affecting performance

Samuel is demonstrating more frustration lately; he is breaking things, occasionally throws things, and seems to pick fights more easily than in prior years.

Samuel hangs on his desk, the teacher's table, and on the walls when standing in line; he frequently lays his head on the desk and wraps his legs around the chairs.

Samuel frequently moves his pencil in his hand, and drops his pencil during classwork.

Adapted from: Dunn, W. (1990). Clinical case workbook I. In C.B. Royeen (Ed.), *AOTA self study series: Assessing function* (Lesson 11). Bethesda, MD: American Occupational Therapy Association. Reprinted with permission.

used to formulate a contextually relevant plan for Samuel in his third grade classroom.

Summary

The evaluation process is the first opportunity that professionals have to demonstrate their skills and respect for the persons being served. It is critical in the current social policy culture, that professionals embrace a person-centered approach to evaluation and intervention planning. Additionally, occupational therapists must take responsibility for understanding the relevance of desired performance in people's lives; this includes evaluating based on performance in the natural contexts for the person being served. We can only know the success of our interventions when we know how the person's actual life has changed.

References

American Occupational Therapy Association. (1994). Uniform terminology for occupational therapy (3rd ed.). *American Journal of Occupational Therapy, 48,* 1047–1054.

American Occupational Therapy Association. (1996). Occupational therapy: A profession in support of full inclusion. *American Journal of Occupational Therapy Association, 50,* 855.

Canadian Association of Occupational Therapists. (1991). Toward outcome measures in occupational therapy. In *Occupational therapy guidelines for client-centered practice.* Toronto, ON: Canadian Association of Occupational Therapists Publications ACE.

Dunn, W. (1990). Clinical case workbook I. In C.B. Royeen (Ed.), *AOTA self study series: Assessing Function.* (Lesson 11). Bethesda, MD: American Occupational Therapy Association.

Dunn, W., Brown, C., McClain, L., & Youngstrom, M. (In press). *The ecology of human performance: Contextual influences on occupational performance.*

Dunn, W., Brown, C., McClain, L., & Westman, K. (1994). The ecology of human performance: A contextual perspective on human occupation. In C.B. Royeen (Ed.), *AOTA self study series: The practice of the future: Putting occupation back into therapy.* (Chapter I). Bethesda, MD: American Occupational Therapy Association.

Dunn, W., Brown, C., & McGuigan, A. (1994). The ecology of human performance: A framework for considering the effect of context. *American Journal of Occupational Therapy, 48(7),* 595–607.

Law, M. (1991). 1991 Muriel Drive lecture. The environment: A focus for occupational therapy. In *Canadian Journal of Occupational Therapy, 58(4),* 171–179.

Law, M., Baptiste, S., Carswell-Opzoomer, A., McColl, M., Polatajko, H., & Pollock, N. (1991). *Canadian Occupational Performance Measure.* Toronto, Canada: Canadian Association of Occupational Therapists Publications.

Letts, L., Law, Rigby, P., Cooper, B., Stewart, D., & Strong, S. (1994). Person-environment assessments in occupational therapy. *American Journal of Occupational Therapy, 48,* 608–618.

Pollock, N. (1993). Client-centered assessment. *American Journal of Occupational Therapy, 47,* 298–301.

Pollock, N., Baptiste, S., Law, M., McColl, M.A., Opzoomer A., & Polatajko, H. (1990). Occupational performance measures: A review based on the guidelines for the client-oriented practice of occupational therapy. *Canadian Journal of Occupational Therapy, 57,* 77–81.

Rosen, M., Clark, G. & Kivits, M. (1976). *The history of mental retardation.* Baltimore: University Park Press.

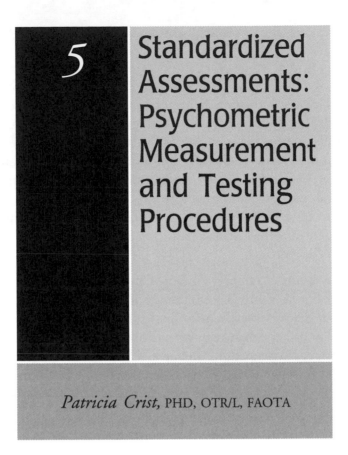

5 Standardized Assessments: Psychometric Measurement and Testing Procedures

Patricia Crist, PHD, OTR/L, FAOTA

Overview

This chapter discusses the importance of psychometric measures for understanding data collected during the evaluation. It identifies the screening process as the beginning point of collecting data. Standardization of assessment is outlined, including psychometrics, basic statistics and measurement theory, reliability and validity of tests, normative data and understanding test scores, and criterion data. Furthermore, it discusses context-specific assessments and the future of standardized assessments in occupational therapy.

Introduction

Accurate, efficient evaluation is an expectation of the trades and professions. The purpose of evaluation is to identify problems needing attention. A consumer would not want a mechanic to begin repairing his or her car before evaluation of a potential problem was completed. A patient would not want to undergo surgery without clear evaluation and identification of an illness or condition needing treatment. Parents do not want to withhold educational services needed for their children to succeed in school, and therefore, request screening for potential developmental or learning deficiencies. Consequently, *no* occupational therapy services should *ever* be instituted under any situation without evaluation information being obtained first. Occupational therapy practitioners have responsibility in selecting the appropriate test, utilizing skilled methods in administering the test to the individual, interpreting the results or scores accurately, and communicating, as well as using, the test results. This responsibility is based on understanding basic psychometric properties related to test and measurement procedures. This chapter provides an introduction to the effective use of tests, regardless of whether the purpose is practice, research, outcomes management, or some other form of accountability or decision-making process.

Evaluation results in not only accurate definition of the problem or performance deficit, but also provides confidence in professional decision-making. Tests are either descriptive, diagnostic, or predictive indicators of significant areas of behavior or performance in given situations. Evaluation is not a waste of time nor money in occupational therapy. What is a waste of time and money in occupational therapy? Without evaluation we risk treating unnecessarily and not being able to provide measured outcomes resulting from occupational therapy services.

The occupational therapist must utilize the assessment process and specific evaluations that are relevant and consistent with the service delivery context and professional competence. The therapist must be aware of the technical adequacy of a testing instrument (including psychometric characteristics), the purpose of and rationale for the test, and the population for which the test is intended (King-Thomas, 1987). The therapist must understand the purpose and value of competent evaluation and must view the process as part of intervention, treatment planning, or research, in order to address individualized needs and monitor progress or change in response to intervention. By understanding basic test and measurement theory and the approaches to the evaluation process presented in this chapter, the occupational therapist will gain knowledge in the essential competencies needed as an evaluator, increase the quality of programming, provide confidence in documented outcomes, while being efficient and able to demonstrate cost effectiveness accurately.

The Evaluation Process: Screening Tools and Assessments

Evaluation is the complex and individually specified process of gathering, interpreting, and reporting information about occupational performance and functional ability. Comprehensive evaluation in occupational therapy requires consideration of the interaction between environmental context and individual performance. For instance, in a recent study, this interaction demonstrated that the outcomes from evaluating a client in the hospital kitchen presented a very different array of performance abilities than when the individual was evaluated in the native (home) environment (Park, Fisher & Velazo, 1994). Both assessment of individual performance abilities and the environmental context in which occupations are performed are essential in occupational therapy assessment procedures, in order to obtain an accurate assessment of both function and dysfunction.

The evaluation process involves:

1) understanding the referral for evaluation, which should identify the desired purpose for the request
2) gathering a history about the individual's prior performance abilities and limitations
3) selecting the appropriate screening or assessment tool
4) adminstering and scoring the test, using published or standardized procedures
5) interpreting the findings
6) effectively communicating the results orally and in writing
7) providing directions for intervention or treatment plans, as well as the ability to predict future performance.

Evaluation is done prior to initiating services, as a measure of performance gains during treatment, throughout service as a formative evaluation of intervention progress, and at the conclusion of intervention to document performance attainment at time of termination. The quality of evaluation outcomes is an interplay between the professional decisions used by the therapist in selecting assessments for the right and specific purpose or need, and the training and knowledge of the evaluator administering the test. Thus, the heart of the assessment process is utilizing evaluations appropriately for the specific situation.

Effective test use requires familiarity with test and measurement construction (Anastasi & Urbina, 1997). This knowledge assists the occupational therapist to evaluate and compare different tests, to choose tests appropriate for the specific situation and individual being evaluated, and to interpret the scores properly.

Assessment tools come in two major types: screening tools and assessments. Screening tools are brief assessment procedures, frequently measuring broad or general performance abilities. Outcomes from the screening process result in identification of performance areas needing additional, more specific, or complex assessment warranting further definition or description. On the other hand, screening may indicate that no problem exists, and so no further assessment is done and no services are instituted. Use of briefer screening tools to identify who needs further evaluation and possible treatment allows efficient use of limited resources, as only those individuals who would benefit from extensive, time-consuming, and therefore, costly additional in-depth evaluation would be so assessed, using only those tests related to performance concerns identified during the screening process.

Methods for collecting information come in the form of assessments. Tools can provide both quantitative and qualitative information for clinical and research purposes. Most importantly, the assessment tool must support the purpose of the evaluation. Several types of tools are utilized in occupational therapy including:

- survey
- observation
- objective rating scale
- inventory
- questionnaire
- interview, activity simulation and performance test, and other electronic or mechanical devices to collect performance or attitude information.

Each of these test types collects different types of information and is considered either standardized or nonstandardized.

Standardized Tests

A standardized test is an evaluation that has undergone rigorous development in order to establish norms for performance, given a comparative sample. A test is a tool to support effective service delivery decisions. Tests, when used appropriately, provide valuable information for intervention planning and monitoring progress; but used inappropriately, they can create severe harm through misidentification, faulty labeling, or misdiagnosis. Uniformity and consistency in administering tests provide accurate assessment of individual abilities, facilitate comparison of performance with others, and enhance communication of evaluation outcomes to other service providers within the continuum of care—even preventing unnecessary re-testing, not to mention providing evidence of prior responsiveness to specific intervention approaches and of therapeutic gains.

Comprehensive, clear instructions for administration and scoring are delineated to ensure uniformity in using the test, session-to-session and evaluator-to-evaluator. Psychometric characteristics, including both reliability and validity, have been studied and are published for reference by the test user. As a result, the evaluator can compare the results on an individual test to a range of performance gathered during one step in the development phase of the instrument, called the process of standardizing or "norming" a test. Norms are derived from empirical studies of expected responses by representative samples of individuals to a given testing condition; these identify both the range and frequency of potential responses for the individual being evaluated. Test development is arduous and costly, but it means that when the test is repeatedly administered to similar individuals, the results will be similar. Standardization procedures, including instructions for evaluation administration and norms, are published in test manuals or professional journals.

The more rigor used in developing and standardizing a test, the more confidence the evaluator can have in the diagnostic or predictive abilities of the test, when used according to published procedures and when comparing individual results with norms appropriate for interpretation. The use of a standardized test determines either current or future client or student capacity or potential. As a result of this testing, the client will have access to needed services and interventions. Thus, a practitioner must be qualified, accurate, and consistent when using assessment procedures.

A standardized test provides specific procedures for administering and scoring the test, in order to ensure uniformity and consistency. The description of specific administration procedures is essential. This information should include a list of the exact materials to be used, exact oral instructions, including how to handle queries from the person being evaluated, demonstration procedures, time limit, and every other response anticipated during the testing procedure. Even pre-testing conditions may be specified, such as avoiding certain foods or activity prior to tests that measure physiological responses. For instances, doing a measure of hyperactivity just after a child's recess or after an adult's consumption of caffeine or other stimulants may distort test results and not be a true or accurate measure of ability or performance competence. Even rate of speaking, tone of voice, position in relation to test situation, voice inflection, and facial expression can all influence test performance.

Standardized Tests versus Standardized Procedures to Assessment

One important criterion for administering any test is for the evaluator to administer the test in a consistent way every time the test is used. All standardized tests describe a specific way to administer the test, which is referred to as *standardized procedures*. Standardized procedures are clearly-delineated, step-by-step instructions for administering an assessment and interpreting results. Standardized procedures remove the variance—called *rater error* or *bias*—in test results, which could be attributed to differences in evaluator skills or performance instead of what is truly desired during measurement—the actual performance of the individual being evaluated. Standardized procedures require training and practice before administration of the test in order to ensure that the evaluator or test administrator implements the exact testing procedures required by the instrument.

Occupational therapy practitioners must realize that, just because a test or evaluation has published extensive standardized procedures, this does not mean that the instrument qualifies as a standardized test. Standardization implies the use of uniform, consistent procedures in administering and scoring a test. Uniformity in procedures means that scores obtained from different evaluators given to the same client would come out the same or be comparable. As a result of using standardized procedures, the performance of the individual being evaluated is being recorded, not the individual attributes or performance inconsistencies of the evaluator. Some tests requires such specific standardized procedures during scoring of the results that certification by the testing company as an evaluator is required prior to use. In other situations, a practitioner may not be able to obtain a test copy unless he or she holds a specific academic degree that should have prepared the individual to use the test correctly. Certification or controlling access to an evaluation increases the likelihood that only qualified individuals are using the assessment and that the test is being used in standardized manner.

Occupational therapists must evaluate a test not only as to how clearly and thoroughly the administration procedures are delineated but also as to how accurate and useful the final scores are. The practitioner must have confidence in the obtained score, due to the diagnostic or predictive uses of the score. Inaccuracy can produce disastrous results. A wrong diagnosis or prediction may deny the patient or client access to valuable interventions, or worse, label the performance ability inaccurately. For instance, a child may be reported to all educators as learning disabled, which will change the quality of interaction and educational expectations. For the appropriately identified child, this is a good outcome. However, if the tests results are inaccurate, the outcome is not a positive one. Practitioners must also be aware of the potentially negative impact of individuals being labeled with a specific problem in some environments. Resources, interactions, and even expectations may change. Thus, ethically, the use of measurement results requires the professional to evaluate the accuracy of a test, as indicated through reported standardization results, as well as to use the test according to standardized procedures. The reader is referred back to Chapters 1 and 11, which discuss ethics in testing, and is encouraged to closely evaluate the psychometric properties of an evaluation before implementation.

Observer or Rater Effects in Testing

The evaluator can influence test results during an evaluation session either by his or her presence or by projecting particular attitudes or expectations into the assessment process. Table 5.1 describes the major sources of rater or observer effects that occur during testing. All create rating error that decreases the measures' reliability and validity. In other words, the rating or score of the client includes some scoring error that can be attributed to the rater or observer and not to the individual being assessed.

The effects of observer or rater bias can be controlled through specific approaches to evaluation. Evaluators should be carefully trained in administering the evaluation and re-checked periodically to ensure that correct procedures are being used. At these times, evaluators can be warned about individual tendencies to rate in a biased manner, in response to characteristics or expectations of the performance being evaluated. Also, the potential influences of their background, presence, or expectations can be reviewed. Routine monitoring is essential to ensure accuracy and that standardized procedures are followed, including responses to inquiries from those being evaluated. In addition, being as unobtrusive as possible during observations is expected in order not to interfere with the performance of the person being evaluated. The most significant strategy, besides periodic re-check on evaluation administration techniques, is to continually be aware of potential sources of observer bias to prevent intrusion of this information creating error in final scores. In cases where known rater bias affected an individual's final performance scores, the occupational therapist is responsible for sharing this in oral and written documentation, as a potential influence on the outcomes from the evaluation process.

A practitioner must be qualified to administer a test. These qualifications are established by the test developer to prevent misuse or abuse in using a specific test. Test manuals will discuss four major aspects of testing that a

■ *Table 5.1.* **Evaluator Effects on Testing**

Observer Bias	
Background Bias	bias attributed to personal background, experiences, or preferences
Errors	
Severity or Leniency	tendency to rate too strictly or too leniently; the reluctance of an evaluator to assess behavior as extreme (severity) or unfavorable (leniency)
Central Tendency	tendency to rate everyone as average performance or towards the middle of the scale in order to avoid extreme scores
Halo Effect	initial impressions, either negative or positive, about the individual affect ratings; a favorable or unfavorable trait not being tested influences test results
Observer Presence	individual changes his or her behavior in response to presence of evaluator
Observer Expectation	evaluator's personal interests and investments are reflected in test results

qualified examiner is able to perform: selection of the test, administration, scoring, and interpretation of scores. Qualification to use a test begins with one's educational background and, in some situations, the allowance or restrictions stated by professional regulation such as certification, licensing, and even specific qualification criteria to administer a test. For instance, in occupational therapy, the *Sensory Integration and Praxis Tests* (SIPT) (Ayres, 1989), the *Functional Independence Measure* (Center for Functional Assessment Research, 1993), and the *Assessment of Motor and Processing Skills* (AMPS) (Fischer, 1992) each have certification procedures that a user must complete prior to being able to use them validly and reliably. On the other hand, a practitioner can become qualified to administer the *Kohlman Evaluation of Living Skills* (KELS) (1992) through careful reading of the manual and practice. In some situations, a test is restricted in use, not to ensure user competence but actually to protect test content and the accurate communication of test information. Regardless of the reason, all practitioners must ensure that they meet the published user qualification criteria, including educational background and test-specific training, before administering and, most importantly, interpreting and planning based on performance outcomes.

Testing conditions are also important and the testing set-up is described carefully in test manuals. Attention must be given to the testing environment, including selection of a suitable testing area that is free from undue noise and distraction and provides adequate seating, ventilation, lighting, and work space for test takers. Attention to these test conditions will ensure increased accuracy in assessment and limit alternative explanations for test performance. Test conditions influence scores by altering performance.

Psychometrics

Test development and standardization approaches described earlier in this chapter mean that the psychometric properties of the test have been studied and published in order to ensure uniformity each time it is used. The user of the test must carefully study and understand not only testing procedures, in order to administer standardized tests properly, but also the psychometric characteristics. Understanding the psychometric qualities of a test requires a fundamental knowledge of statistics and the basic approaches used to demonstrate the "goodness" of a test, called *reliability* and *validity*. One of the most important aspects of a well-standardized test is the rigorous testing to establish the assessment's reliability and validity, in order to interpret results accurately and consistently. A test is only as good as its reported psychometric properties.

Tables 5.2 through 5.5 outline basic concepts related to test statistics, measurement theory, reliability, and validity. Each of these concepts could be discussed extensively. For purposes of this chapter, they will only be

■ *Table 5.2.* **Basic Statistics Used to Report Test Standardization**

Statistics	the use of math principles and equations to describe a characteristic or draw inferences by summarizing quantitative data;
Normal Distribution	the use of a normal, bell-shaped curve that has the largest number of responses in the center of the curve, is symmetrical, and the number drops off in each direction;
Mean	a measure of central tendency which describes average group or individual performance; symbol − x;
Standard Deviation	specific, gradually decreasing areas or regions marked off under the normal curve, starting at the center of the curve, which subdivide scores that vary from the mean or central tendency; 68.26% of the curve is within the area of ± 1 SD (or 34.13% on one side only); ± 2 SD = 95.44% and ± 3 SD = 99.72% symbol = SD;
Correlation	the degree of relationship between two variables; does not imply causality, but does imply association;
Correlation Coefficient	a numerical index stating the degree of correlation or relationship between two variables; The coefficient ranges from + 1.0 to − 1.0. A positive correlation coefficient means if the individual's score is high on one variable, the other is high whereas a negative correlation means is inverse, a high score on one variable means a low one on the other; symbol = r;
Level of Significance	identifies the probability that chance influences the results or outcomes. The lower the level, the less confidence in the results; typically, the probability for confidence must be .05 or better, which indicates that the probability of a given result occurring by chance is less than 5 out of 100; symbol = p.

introduced for entry-level practitioners to refer to when examining any test they are considering or in interpreting individual results following administration.

BASIC STATISTICS AND MEASUREMENT THEORY

The development, selection, and use of standardized tests require a fundamental understanding of statistics and measurement theory. Frequently-used terms in test manuals or reviews are introduced in Tables 5.2 and 5.3. *Norms* are the normative data in a specific test. A *correlation* is a specific statistical procedure frequently used in reliability studies for tests. *Correlation coefficients* report the amount two variables have in common. Reliability coefficients in tests must be .8 or higher to be considered satisfactory. The *level of significance* is used in normative studies to detect differences in performance between two groups on one variable. The ability to predict differences is identified and reported as probability. Reports will state: p = a number or p ≤ a number that is an outcome of a statistical test, including correlations. Readers are encouraged to review statistical processes in other sources if these terms are unfamiliar, as only a brief review is possible here.

■ *Table 5.3.* **Fundamental Measurement Concepts**

Error of Measurement	the difference between the real score of an individual and the observed score during one session; error is introduced through various forms of bias and inability to use the test as designed
Item Bias	the relative difficulty of an individual test item for groups with cultural or experimental backgrounds different from the normative population
Rater Error	error introduced by evaluators when they do not use standardized procedures published for a test or introduce observer/evaluator effects into the testing situation
Individual Error	the individual does something either prior to or during the testing situation which introduces error
Standard Error of Measurement	the degree that an individual score will deviate from the true score as a result of irrelevant or chance occurrences as well as sources of error in measurement; expresses the reliability of individual scores and the optimal test environment; noted in test manuals as SEM
Standard Error of Estimate	the degree of predictive validity or margin of error expected in a person's criterion score; expresses the validity of a test; noted in test manuals as SE_{est}
Reliability Coefficient	the coefficient tells the portion of score variance that is not attributed to error in testing; perfect agreement = 1.0 and is the expression of the degree of reliability, called stability, offered by a test; "the possibility of a test giving the same results in identical testing circumstances"; the SEM
Validity Coefficient	the correlation between a test score and each criterion as a calculation of test validity ranges from 0 to 1.00; rarely will the coefficient exceed 60; "the degree the test measures what it is supposed to"; the Se_{est}
Intra-Individual Score Differences	the reliability (SEM) between two scores for the same individual at different times; SE_{diff}.

Any individual score on one evaluation is a combination of the individual's true score plus error contributing to the final score:

Current Score = True Score + Testing Error

The goal in administering tests is to decrease, control, or eliminate sources of testing error, so that the evaluator can have confidence that the test score of performance observation is an estimate of the individual's real abilities and not influenced by other explanations. Decreasing error increases the precision or stability of a test or individual test results. If error is large, then the reliability of an individual test score or a test itself is challenged. For instance, the *standard error of measurement* (SEM), frequently reported as the score ± SEM, expresses the degree of confidence one can have that an individual score will fall within the stated region, and safeguards against placing undue emphasis on a single score from a single situation. In testing, the smallest SEM possible is desired and is positively influenced by the increased reliability of a test

■ *Table 5.4.* **Methods for Determining Reliability in Tests**

Test-Retest	a measure of test score stability on the same version of the test repeated over two occasions; based on a correlation of the scores obtained during each of two administrations; useful for tools monitoring change over time
Intrarater Reliability	consistency in measurement and scoring by the evaluator when two test results from two similar situations are correlated
Interrater or Interobserver Reliability	the degree of agreement between the scores from two raters following observation and rating of the same subject; correlations of .85 or higher are expected to compare the objective competency between two raters of the same testing condition
Alternate or Parallel Forms	useful when multiple, equivalent forms of the same test are needed; particularly useful when one responds to the earlier test items can easily be recalled and influence the responses on the second test after a lapse of time (alternate); while the forms contain different questions, similar items on each test are expected to have item equality, making the tests equal at a given point in time (parallel); correlation should be >.80
Internal Consistency	reflects the degree of homogeneity between test items; items measure the same construct; correlation should be >.80
Split Half	the results from performance on the first half of the test are correlated with the second half or the scores on all even-numbered items are compared to odd-numbered ones
Covariance Procedures	the average of all split-half tests; expressed as KR20 or KR21; the consistency of response between all items on a test; referred to as interitem consistency

itself. *Reliability* is the accuracy and stability of a measure, whereas *validity* is how well a test measures what it purports to measure. Validity is the meaning of a test. Understanding statistics related to measurement theory is important when selecting and interpreting test results.

RELIABILITY AND VALIDITY IN TESTING

Reliability and validity are the two most important concepts arising from psychometric or measurement theory. Tables 5.4 and 5.5 introduce the primary types of reliability and validity that are essential to understand in the selection and utilization of a test for clinical or research purposes.

Reliability refers to the consistency between scores obtained by the same individual on different occasions, with equivalent sets of items or other testing conditions (Anastasi, 1988). Reliability is the extent to which a test captures an individual's true score, as a result of limited error possibilities.

Error results when there is a breakdown in uniform testing conditions such as the testing environment, method of giving instructions and answering queries by the person being evaluated, time limits, rapport, and other influ-

■ *Table 5.5.* Methods for Determining Validity in Tests

Face Validity	from appearance, and without statistical proof, the test items appear to address the purpose of the test and the variables to be measured; subjective, logical judgment by the author or experts on the topic
Content Validity	the items on a test represent a sufficient, representative sample of the domain or construct being examined; requires selection of a specific aspect of the behavioral domain evaluated; designed to measure the level of mastery of a particular content domain
Criterion-Related Validity	the ability to determine performance on one test based on the performance on another test; the degree of agreement between two tests; determines the accuracy of prediction which is obtained by squaring the validity coefficient (r^2), which tells us how much variance the predictor variable is able to explain
Concurrent or Congruent Validity	the extent of agreement between two simultaneous measures of the same behaviors or traits
Predictive Validity	the extent of agreement between the current test results and a future assessment; used to make predictions about future behavior
Construct Validity	based on the theoretical framework to test the "goodness-of-fit" between the theorized construct and resulting data from a test; a gauge of the ability of a test to measure a trait or hypothesis that is not observable
Convergent Validity	the test results should correlate highly with another measure of the same variable or construct; infer degree of agreement measuring the same trait with two different tests of the same trait or construct
Discriminant Validity	the test results should not correlate with another measure of the same variable or construct; infer degree of disagreement measuring the same trait with two different tests of the same trait or construct
Factorial Validity	the identification of interrelated behaviors, abilities, or functions in an individual that contribute to collective abilities or functions; correlation of the test with other group to define the common traits it measures

ences. Reliability is always reported using a correlation statistic to determine consistency or agreement between testing situations. *Test-retest reliability* determines the degree of variance in responses when the same test is given to the same individual across a sufficient period of time that the individual cannot remember his or her responses to items between the two testing times. However, time lapse is short enough that the variable being measured would not have changed. Typically, around 2 weeks lapse between the first and second administration of the same test. *Interrater* and *intrarater reliability* are important to control for error attributed to scorer performance. Training and experience in the use of standardized procedures control for this source of error. *Alternate-form reliability* avoids test-retest reliability as the same person can be tested immediately with two equivalent forms of the same test; item sampling and content sampling are two important components of alternate-form reliability. Error in this form of reliability is attributed to fluctuations in performance on one set of items compared to another set. *Split-half reliability* assesses the consistency of content between two forms of the test. *Covariance procedures* are a measure of interitem consistency or homogeneity. This reliability weakens as interitem heterogeneity increases.

In summary, test-retest and alternate-form (delayed) are problematic for time sampling error. Alternate-form (immediate and delayed), split-half, Kuder-Richardson (KR20 and 21), and coefficient alpha introduce the potential for content sampling error with the later type of reliability and also contribute error through content heterogeneity. Interrater and intrarater reliability is dampened by error attributed to interscorer or intrascorer differences.

Validity tells us what construct, trait, or behavior the test score measures. The most powerful form of validity is predictive ability. Predictive validity allows practitioners to take performance or functional measures now and project the likely outcomes following intervention, given the current abilities of the individual being tested. Validity supports the correct interpretation of obtained scores from an evaluation session. Most statistical studies of validity of a specific test report using forms of measurement reliability to determine the various forms of validity reported in Table 5.5.

Before leaving this section, one must ask two timeless questions: Can a test have good reliability but poor validity? Can a test have good validity with poor reliability? The answers demonstrate one's understanding of these two psychometric concepts. Establishing the validity of tests is more important than reliability, as validity is a check frequently against some established external criterion demonstrating that the test measures whatever it is designed to measure (Anatasi & Urbina, 1997). The validity coefficient of a test enables the test user to assess how well the individual test results or score compare to a criterion measure. For instance, when occupational therapists assess muscle strength or handwriting, they look at the validity of the test in measuring the desired performance and not at some other undesirable aspect contributing to performance.

Norms and Understanding Test Scores

In order to properly use and interpret test results, the occupational therapy practitioner must understand four additional concepts: norms, types of scores, rating scale types, and item analysis. *Norms* are the test performance of the standardization sample (Anastasi & Urbina, 1997). *Types of scores or scales* allow the comparison of an individual score with the standardization sample. The *type of rating scale* determines the performance information obtained from an evaluation. *Item analysis* provides both qualitative information, in terms of content and form, and quantitative information regarding the utility and accuracy of a specific item on a test. Each of these concepts is discussed briefly below and a table is provided to describe related terminology. These allow the practitioner to understand and apply test results for both clinical and research purposes. Treatment planning and results from research can be no better than the psychometric properties of the test used to measure individual performance or service delivery outcomes.

NORMS

The conversion of an individual's raw score on a test is only relevant when compared to other similar individuals, referred to as *normative groups* or *norms*. For instance, when evaluating an individual's sensory processing deficits following a stroke, the occupational therapist must select a test that was standardized on a similar population. Using a test of sensory processing problems developed for children with sensory integrative function, even though the same global problem is measured, is not appropriate, because the same sensory deficit may vary because of developmental variances or in response to different pathological conditions causing the problem. Using published norms based on persons with similar characteristics or performance problems supports the practitioner in making a determination of the amount of ability or disability evidenced by the person evaluated. Norms are based on statistical procedures applied to a large sample of results gathered from a group of individuals. In Table 5.6, a brief review of fundamental statistical concepts relevant to test and measurements procedures is provided.

Types of Scores and Scales

Raw scores acquired from the performance of an individual on a test usually must be converted to some scale or format that gives interpretative meaning to the score. The raw score is compared to a normative sample or fixed reference group.

Table 5.7 lists several traditional ways in which a raw score is converted to another form in order to "place" the individual's performance within that of a group of individuals with similar characteristics. Use of standard scores not only enhances communication, as scores are transformed to a traditional scale used by many tests, but these other approaches also permit comparison of performance across several tests, as the normal curve is a common referent point for all, as seen in Figure 5.1a. This enhances communication of different test results for an individual.

Additionally, transforming raw scores to standard scores permits different occupational therapy practitioners or members of an interdisciplinary service delivery team, each of whom may have evaluated an individual using different

■ *Table 5.6.* Norms and Related Measurement Concepts

Raw Score	an individual's score on a test before the score is converted to a comparison scale or normative information
Frequency Distribution	a tabulation of raw scores into a table or graph to represent grouping of scores into intervals or total tallies
Normal Curve	a mathematically-determined curve representing group scores with the mean, median, and mode at the same center point (unimodal); the curve is bell-shaped and bilaterally symmetrical
Norms	the reported test performance of individuals with specific demographic characteristics in the standardization sample
Normative Sample	the standardization group
Developmental Norms	standardization of group scores reflecting developmental sequence or stages; frequently age-equivalents are stated so that individual performance can be compared to the normative sample
National Anchor Norms	the normative data reflect the normal distribution curve and allows comparison of individual performance on a test by referring to how far the score deviates from the mean and is stated in terms of standard deviations
Fixed Reference Group	a nonnormative scale utilizing a specific group in order to ensure comparability of an individual score with a sample of scores from a group of individuals with similar demographics
Mental Age	standardization sample based on mental level or capacity
Grade Equivalents	standardization sample based on performance expectations at different levels of schooling
Measures of Central Tendency *Mean (M)*	the average score calculated by totaling all scores and dividing the sum by the number of cases (N)
Median	middle-most score when all scores have been arranged in order of size (small to large)
Mode	most frequent score
Measures of Variability	also referred to as measures of dispersion
Standard Deviation (SD)	how far each score varies from the mean; permits an individual score to be referenced within a norm group for comparative purposes, by the distance the score is from the mean
Variance	how far each score varies from the median; also called the mean square deviation
Range	range between the lowest and highest scores within a group of scores

■ *Table 5.7.* Types of Scores and Scales

Profile	reporting form for individual test scores that understandably compares individual performance to the standardization across several tests of subtests from one evaluation
Percentile Score	an individual's score is expressed as the percentage of those who fall below an individual's raw score on a scale; the 50th percentile corresponds with the median
Percentile Rank	a score for an individual is stated in terms of the percentage of other scores that fall below an individual's raw score on a scale; 50th percentile corresponds with median
Deviation Score	conversion of mental age scores to uniform index reflecting the relative intelligence in relationship to chronological age; expressed as a median of 100 + one standard deviation; a standard deviation on the *Stanford-Binet (SB)* is 16 and on the *College Entrance Examination Board (CEEB)* is 15; sometimes this is called the deviation IQ and is represented by 100+16 (SB) or 100+15 (CEEB)
Standard Score	a derived score that expresses an individual's score in terms of distance from the mean
z-score	an individual's score is expressed using the standard deviation from the mean of the normative sample; expressed as the mean ±1 standard deviation
t-score	an individual score is normalized with 50 representing the mean of the standardization group and ±10 the standard deviation; expressed as 50±10
Stanine	an individual's score is transformed into a score ranging from 1 to 9 with a mean of 5 and ±2 standard deviation approximately; expressed as 5±~2

tests for similar problems, to compare results. Thus, using standard scores or other types of score transformation methods supports the practitioner in determining how much of a problem, issue, or characteristic is present, compared to normative samples or across several tests of the same individual.

In closing, a profile may or may not use standard score transformations. A profile does provide a carefully planned report of results, so that the user, whether a practitioner, teacher, or parent, can access easily information.

Rating Scale Types

Occupational therapy practitioners elicit self-reporting data, attitudinal questionnaires, and surveys frequently to determine intervention effectiveness, but more importantly, during program evaluation. While these forms of assessment appear easy to set up and administer, the type of rating scale used will determine the effectiveness of the tool. To create a quality survey or attitude scale that is valid can be very time-consuming, and for that reason, using a widely published test is better than inventing one's own. Second, the scale selected can determine the value of the information obtained for future treatment planning or research interpretation. Thus, a basic understanding

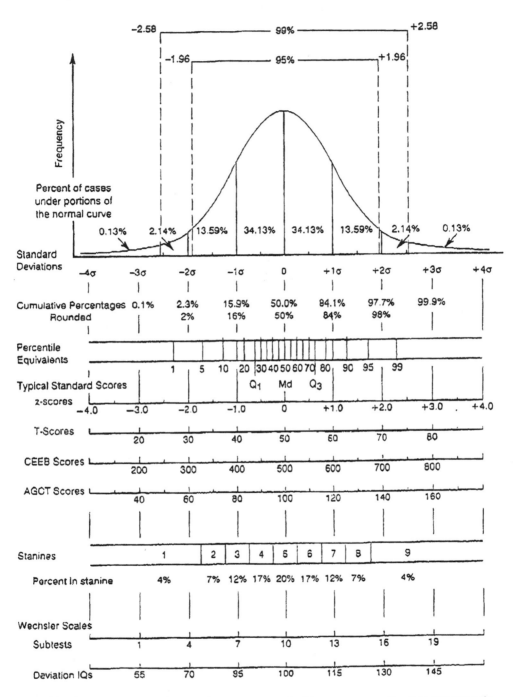

Note: This chart cannot be used to equate scores on one text to scores on another test. For example, both 600 on the CEEB and 120 on the AGCT are one standard deviation above their respective means, but they do not represent "equal" standings because the scores were obtained from different groups.

Figure 5.1. Characteristics of the normal curve. *Note.* Based on data from the *Test Service Bulletin* No. 48, January, 1955 of The Psychological Corporation. Reprinted with permission. All rights reserved.

of different rating scales types is essential in order for a person to be an effective evaluator.

For instance, giving a middle point in a rating scale allows a responder not to make a choice about how he or she really feels about an issue. Not giving a middle point, forces the responder to make a choice. While "fence-sitting" is typically a preferred, less stress-producing event for persons taking the test, no real descriptive information is obtained. Since most persons, given indecision, will "fence-sit" on especially challenging or threatening issues, the evaluator loses valuable information. On the other hand, not giving a middle point may cause a person to refuse to rate or respond and may even lead him or her to discontinue the evaluation session prematurely.

Common rating scale types are reported in Table 5.8, as an introduction to this psychometric area. In these scales, the respondent is indicating his or

■ *Table 5.8.* **Rating Scale Types and Other Methods for Evaluation**

Rating Scales	provides mechanism to gather strength of response or feeling
Likert	a scale that expresses type of response to an item; for instance, using the categories: strongly agree; agree; undecided; disagree; strongly disagree
Guttman	provides an ordered set of items with increasing strength of response; the point at which responders can no longer agree with the statement is considered an indication of how much they agree or disagree with an attitude, issue, or characteristic
Thurstone	the respondent's score is the median value including only statements that are endorsed
Other Measurement Scales	
Checklist	can give wide coverage to a complex variable or construct using either a present-absent format (for instance, "Check those that describe your work abilities from the following list of characteristics: ___organized; ___flexible; ___self-directed"; or multiple choice format (for instance, "quality of work: excellent ___; average ___; poor ___")
Forced Choice	attempts to reduce bias in response, as must choose best among items that are both probable (for instance, "indicate the degree which the following statement describes your interest); very much or just a little: ___reading novels in spare time")
Semantic Differential	subjective evaluation of concepts in terms of evaluation of "goodness" ("good-bad; fair-unfair"); potency or strength of response ("heavy-light, hard-soft") or activity dimensions ("active-passive; exciting-dull"); will have multi-point scale with these concepts as anchor on the continuum, so that responder can indicate preference)
Q-sort	responder is given a list of items to sort according to an established criterion and sorting of these items is studied or evaluated (for instance, you ask the person to sort a stack of behaviors into three piles: "current activities; would like to learn; and prefer never to do")

her level of agreement or disagreement with the statement given. These response scales have been tested rigorously both from the theoretical and statistical standpoints, which are beyond the scope of this discussion. Just as important as the rating scale selected, is the meaningfulness of the descriptor being rated. Selection of valid or relevant attitudes, self-report, or survey items is essential. The rule is, "Only ask what you need to know about," whether for research, service delivery, or program planning purposes.

Several errors are discussed in relation to interpreting evaluation outcomes from a rating:

- *Generosity error* occurs when the individual tends to give responses a more favorable or disfavorable rating than deserved.
- *Ambiguity error* is when the rater's interpretation of an item varies from the interpretation others raters may possess.
- *Halo effect* is when one's opinion strongly influences overall impressions.
- *Central tendency error* is the tendency to avoid extreme responses.
- *Leniency or severity error* is the tendency to avoid unfavorable ratings or to be just the opposite, too easy; sometimes referred to as *extreme score error.*
- *Proximity error* is when an event immediately preceding the event to be rated influences the rating.
- *Logical error* occurs when there is an inappropriate or insufficient opportunity to observe the behavior being rated.
- *Contrast error* occurs when there is a marked difference between the characteristics of the rater and the person or item being rated.

The influence of these various errors can be controlled by the occupational therapist by ensuring adequate training in a technique, following established protocol, including good instructions to the person being evaluated, and constant awareness that these sources of error can influence information obtained through rating scales—in general, follow good test administration procedures and the ratings obtained will be more accurate.

ITEM ANALYSIS

Understanding item analysis can help the occupational therapist select and use published tests or evaluate responses on computer-scored assessments such as quizzes, midterms, and surveys. Certainly the validity and reliability of any test depends ultimately on the quality of the items in a test. Several approaches to item analysis are defined in Table 5.9. The simplest form of item analysis is item difficulty. Reflective evaluators will not stop at this point to decide whether a question is good or not; they will also look at how well the item differentiates persons who perform similarly on both the item and the overall

■ *Table 5.9.* Item Analysis

Item Difficulty	typically, the difficulty of an item is defined in terms of the percentage or proportion of answers correct, and contributes to the overall difficulty of the whole test
Item Discrimination	refers to the degree that an item differentiates correctly what the test is designed to measure; traditionally this process compares the individual responses on one item to the overall performance of these individuals on the test; good item discrimination means that an individual who scored best on the test got it right, while a person who scored worst on the test, got it wrong; if this does not happen, then a question's discrimination index will be lower, as the question does not differentiate performance accurately—in other words, more individuals in a group who answered the item correctly, did not make the higher grades in the class, or vice versa
Cross-Validation	the process of comparing the responses on a set of questions obtained from one group to the responses to the same set of questions by a totally different but similar group, to see whether the same results are obtained
Rasch Analysis	this item analysis reflects the performance ability of the person tested, the item difficulty, the severity of the rater in scoring the specific performance of the person being evaluated, and the challenge or degree of difficulty of the evaluation task used to measure the desired performance or behavior.

test, using a correlation. Computer scoring packages are available to easily perform an item discrimination analysis for each item. Thus, an evaluator only eliminates test items with low item discrimination correlations, as the question was answered by both the highest and lowest performers in the class in the same way, preventing the individual item from being a good discriminator.

Test construction is a science in itself but approaches such as cross validation, and others beyond the scope of this text, provide a way to both qualitatively and quantitatively assess an item on a test. Tests constructed using the Rasch Model of measurement are emerging as a respected approach to item development in occupational therapy. Using this method in occupational therapy is very relevant in order to measure complex behavior that is highly variant, especially when rating observed performance during activities and tasks with specific performance components or categories. Fisher (1995) states that the Rasch Model in occupational therapy can be used to express performance as a function of the ability of that person, the skill item difficulty, severity of the rater, and the challenge of the task performed. From a test validity perspective, this approach to item development in occupational therapy is a complex procedure, but it is an emerging approach that holds great promise for the skills and activities evaluated in occupational therapy.

Norm-Referenced and Criterion-Referenced Testing Approaches

Two primary approaches to testing are available: norm-referenced testing and criterion-referenced testing. *Norm-referenced testing* uses known population parameters as a standard to describe occupational performance. *Criterion-referenced testing,* frequently also called *mastery testing,* uses a specific content domain or functional levels to describe occupational performance. Criterion-referenced testing measures the degree to which an individual has achieved mastery in skills or abilities.

The reason for using one approach or the other depends on the purpose for measuring an individual's performance in occupational therapy. The occupational therapist must, first, decide how he or she wishes to define or describe the performance ability being measured and the purpose for doing an evaluation, before selecting an appropriate evaluation instrument.

NORM-REFERENCED APPROACH

The essential feature of norm-referenced assessment is the interpretation of test results in terms of norms. A norm is the normal or average performance. The objective of the norm-referenced test is to compare ratings of individual performance to a larger, similar, comparative sample, using test items from a standardized evaluation. The outcome is the ability to evaluate an individual test score in relationship to the group used to establish the norms for the test, called the *standardization sample.* This sample establishes the norms that are used to evaluate the individual's score, in terms of how much above or below average it is. Norms permit the abilities of the individual to be compared to the normative or standardization sample. Norms provide a comparison of the range of possible scores, rather than simply show the presence or absence of a characteristic, ability, or skill, as criterion-referenced approaches do.

While not using a standardized test per se, many professors in their classes provide statistical information, including the class average score (the mean) and the variation in performance (standard deviation) for the combined class. This permits the individual to compare his or her own performance to what other class members were able to achieve. The instructor uses this information to assign a letter grade, interpreting the results to mean that the person who scored the highest on the test knew the most and assigning the lowest grade to the person who demonstrated he or she knew the least, as indicated by scores on the test. While the typical college test is not considered to be standardized, this same process is how scores are compared using a rigorously developed standardized test. A standardized test is only as good as the procedures used to develop it, including the establishment of norms, standardized procedures, and studies of the "goodness" of the test, referred to as the *psychometric characteristics* of the test or assessment.

An occupational therapy practitioner will use a norm-referenced test when he or she wants to establish the degree of ability or disability, function or dysfunction, adaptation or maladaptation, health or illness of individual performance in relationship to the normative sample. For instance, the practitioner may want to establish the degree of short-term memory that is present, compare an individual's grip strength to that of others with similar characteristics, or assess a child's ability to sustain attention during an activity in relationship to others with a similar diagnosis or age. In order to make this comparison, the practitioner must first determine how similar the individual client is to the individuals in the normative sample. Characteristics that influence performance or the condition should be used to decide whether individual performance on the assessment can be compared with the norm group. Characteristics such as age, gender, occupation, diagnosis, time since onset of injury or illness, stage or level of disability, and even coexisting conditions are some of the potential issues to be considered before use and interpretation of individual scores. All individual deviations from the normative sample affect the reliability and validity of the test and must be reported when interpreting tests, as these may influence test results.

Norm-referenced tests are frequently employed when measuring individual response to intervention over a period of time, to assess changes in function or ability. Use of norm-referenced assessments also provides a target range for typical or expected performance abilities, to determine when treatment can be discontinued. In order to use a test to determine treatment outcomes or when to conclude intervention, the test must have been developed for these purposes and the psychometric information must provide validity and reliability information to substantiate this type of use. Not every norm-referenced test can be used to repeatedly measure response to occupational therapy interventions. Some can be used only once to identify the relative degree of dysfunction present.

CRITERION-REFERENCED APPROACH

The prominent characteristic of criterion-referenced assessment is its interpretation of test performance in terms of content meaning or mastery (Anastasi, 1988). The objective of the test is to find out what test takers can do and what they know, not how they compare with others. Several alternative terms exist for criterion-referenced assessments: domain-referenced, content-referenced, and objective-referenced. These terms can be used interchangeably, but the use of the term criterion-referenced is the most popular. This method is used when the content, either skills or information, can be clearly delineated in behavioral terms and, preferably, in sequential performance steps or learning objectives. Since testing items sample each step or objective, criterion-referenced methods are best used to test essential, fundamental skills and abilities, in highly structured situations.

Mastery testing is used to indicate whether the individual has or has not attained a specified level of ability. Mastery testing is used in measuring chosen objectives in practical situations, after specific individualized training: for example, lab practical examinations in school or skill demonstrations in the clinic. Mastery testing yields an all-or-none score, mastered or nonmastered. Therefore, a specific cut-off score, frequently referred to as a "cut score," must be established prior to testing. A "cut score" can be established through empirical comparative testing or as a judgment regarding what skill or performance competence level indicates sufficient mastery of the desired content or skill.

An occupational therapist might use a criterion-referenced evaluation to see whether a client has mastered a specific dressing activity or to identify the number of safety hazards the client can identify in his or her home, the level of cognitive ability a person demonstrates, or the chances of achieving an expected level of performance following therapy, based on current activity skills or competencies. Computer-assisted, self-paced learning designed for consumer education programs, or more recently, use of treatment protocols, frequently utilize criterion-referenced assessment procedures. In both these learning situations, criterion-referenced items can be used to identify a specific performance difficulty, to identify prerequisite skills, to acquire the performance skills then in deficit, and to prescribe particular intervention procedures. These procedures are useful as outcome measures for intervention processes, as well as quality improvement indicators during program evaluation. In occupational therapy education, criterion-referenced assessments are frequently used to assess student skill acquisition related to specific evaluations and intervention approaches. During fieldwork Level II, the evaluation instrument is criterion-referenced, as the criteria stated in the national fieldwork evaluation are utilized to assess the student's level of mastery in relationship to identified competency requirements for entry level practice skills (Cooper & Crist, 1988). The national certification examination is also a criterion-referenced test. In school-based practice, occupational therapists are familiar with competency-based education, which uses criterion-referenced performance targets.

COMPARISON BETWEEN APPROACHES

In reality, the normative approach underlies all testing (Nitko, 1984; Anastasi, 1988). In occupational therapy, knowledge regarding performance is related to expected skill acquisition patterns from a developmental, behavioral, or educational perspective. Our standard for measuring all performance is based on ability continuums derived from assumptions and information about how other individuals would perform in similar situations or contexts. Mastery or criterion-referenced approaches do not ignore individual differences, but simply set a specific cut-off score to divide performance into one of two categories such as acquired and not acquired, competent or not competent, able or unable. This cut-off is established by using knowledge to decide when a specific criterion or level of performance is mastered.

The problem with criterion-referenced testing is that information regarding individual differences is lost, as the person either "meets" or "does not meet" the established criterion. However, criterion-referenced testing is beneficial in occupational therapy when a practitioner wants to ensure that specific or minimal competence in performing a specific activity or occupation is present for decision-making purposes. For instance, if the occupational therapist must determine when a client is able to live in a specific community environment, such as his or her own home or a supported living environment, criterion-referenced evaluations are appropriate to ensure that the client has the minimal competencies required for successful or safe living in the specific situation.

The benefit of using norm-referenced testing in occupational therapy is that the occupational therapist can determine the degree of specific skill acquisition or performance competence for each individual and compare this data to a set of normed performance expectations. Descriptions of performance or activity abilities are very specific and can be compared to developmental or hierarchical skill acquisition expectations. An individual's degree of ability or disability can be compared to well-established standards regarding a specific content or performance domain. For instance, norm-referenced testing is beneficial in occupational therapy, when the practitioner wants to measure ongoing responses or outcomes to the treatment or intervention process, such as when trying to measure range of motion increases resulting across several treatment sessions or the level of cognitive ability a client is utilizing in order to select appropriate activities.

Thus, while norm- and criterion-referenced assessments both reflect normative expectations to some degree, the selection of a specific evaluation must include both the performance to be measured and the purpose for doing the evaluation. Norm-referenced assessment compares an individual's abilities to a group of similar persons, whereas criterion-referenced assessment identifies the degree to which an individual has mastered a well-defined competency or performance objective. Norm-referenced assessment is designed to measure variability or differences among individuals, whereas criterion-referenced measurement measures competence in successive skill performance.

Context-Specific Testing, Including Ecological Assessment

With the introduction of *Uniform Terminology for Occupational Therapy, 3rd ed.* (AOTA, 1994), the environment became a mediating variable in determining individual occupational performance abilities. For instance, the results from an activities-of-daily-life assessment may differ markedly if the individual is tested in the clinic rather than in his or her own home where he or she is familiar with resources, spatial organization, and environmental cues. The quality of one's occupational performance is influenced by characteristics of the environment, age, disability status, and temporal considerations. For instance, an individual who uses a wheelchair for mobility becomes increasingly disabled if automatic door openers are not available, if curb cuts are not present, or if a building has front entrance steps without access to a ramp or elevator for access. Context-specific testing is essential in occupational therapy to determine discharge readiness and approaches utilized already and additional ones needed to enhance independent performance.

Authentic assessment (McCowan, Driscoll, & Roop, 1995) is used to assess problem-solving and critical thinking in real-life contexts. These types of tests are used to measure complex performance.

Ecological assessment as a type of context-specific assessment was introduced to evaluate the individual and the environment as a single unit and to provide a broad perspective on performance within a given environment (Thomas & Hacker, 1987). Ecological assessment refers to measures that are gathered within a specific environment or with a specific environment or situation in mind. Observations, histories, interviews, checklists, and questionnaires are aspects of ecological assessment.

Identification of Evaluations

Occupational therapy practitioners are advised to carefully consider the background used to establish the standardization of an evaluation and are cautioned to use each test according to its intended purpose. This requirement increases the degree of accuracy and confidence in interpreting results and limits negative outcomes. Furthermore, a therapist should carefully consider the appropriateness of using a standardized test or part of the test outside its original context or testing sequence. When using a test in situations other than those for which it was intended, such as using a sensorimotor test standardized for children on adults, one should not report scores. Such data should be reported descriptively. Lastly, significant caution, almost avoidance, should be exercised in creating one's own situation-specific diagnostic, predictive, or performance capacity evaluations without undertaking standardization in order to ensure reliability and validity.

Occupational therapy practitioners recognize that access to standardized assessments poses one of our greatest professional dilemmas for both clinical and research applications. As a result, the American Occupational Therapy Foundation (1996) has undertaken the development of assessments relevant to occupational therapy concerns, as a major research objective. More dedicated test development is needed in occupational therapy.

In the meantime, practitioners must select and use tests wisely by reviewing carefully the instrument's objectives, standardization, and application before using. Training in administering the assessment is essential. Several widely utilized measurement references are available in major libraries to initially review information about major standardized tests: the *Mental Measurement Yearbooks (MMY)*; *Tests in Print by Buros*; *Test Collection Biographies*, by the Educational Testing Service; *Tests in Microfiche*, distributed by Test Collection, ETS. Besides these major sources, a vast store of unpublished tests is described or reproduced in books, journals, and unpublished reports. Almost every profession has specific books published reviewing commonly used professional evaluations. For instance, in occupational therapy, books like *Occupational Therapy Assessment Tools: An Annotated Index* (2nd ed.) (Asher, 1996) and *The Evaluative Process in Psychiatric Occupational Therapy* (Hemphill, 1982) have been published.

Obtaining copies of test manuals and evaluations is essential. Contacting assessment authors or test publishers is one of the best ways to do this. Also, many of the references above will list addresses of the publishers. An individual can request a sample of the test, called a *specimen set*, to evaluate the test for specific applications before purchasing. The test manual should provide the essential information for administration, scoring, and interpretation of scores. Detailed instructions, a scoring key, and norms should be identified. The manual should report the description and number of individuals and methods used to establish the norms, reliability, and validity of the test.

More recently, electronic library resources are emerging to assist with identification of tests and measurements. Two examples are *Health and Psycho-social Instruments (HaPI)* and the World Wide Web. *HaPI* is a CD-ROM database designed to provide access to information on measurement instruments in the areas of health and behavioral sciences. *HaPI* currently contains 42,000 records and continues to grow. *HaPI* indexes unpublished and recently developed surveys, questionnaires, and other qualitative and quantitative tools. The database includes instruments of all types, including conventional, non-traditional, and innovative methods. The actual instruments are not on the database. *HaPI* includes references and abstracts to journal articles, books, and other publications with information about tools. Most important to practitioners, researchers, and students, *HaPI* has a "document delivery service" that allows the individual to obtain copies of the instrument with permission pre-obtained from the author for clinical or research use. The agency overseeing *HaPI* will provide information regarding the development, reliability, and validity of the instrument. The World Wide Web (WWW) or Internet is becoming a quick way to access information on published evaluations. In fact, many web sites offer information regarding the test and even allow users to download a test sample to try it out before purchase. Easy ordering information is provided as well as sources to consult for additional questions. Caution is recommended in placing a credit card order using the Internet at this time, as it can be accessed publicly and abused.

The Future of Standardized Evaluation in Occupational Therapy

A STARTING POINT

This chapter on basic psychometric concepts used in test and measurements is only an introduction to use of tests for entry-level practitioners. These properties will assist practitioners in becoming initially familiar with the "goodness" of a specific test for a specific use and determining how much confidence can be placed on the accuracy of the results. Hopefully, with this chapter as a reference, initial understanding of information contained in test manuals, as well as journal publications exploring specific psychometric properties, will be clearer. All practitioners are required to understand the psychometric characteristics and findings related to every test they administer. Only then can the therapists or researcher communicate the results of the tests confidently and ethically. The problems of misidentification or even mislabeling as a result of test outcomes are costly both to the consumers we serve, but also to service delivery, including faulty outcomes management, service inefficiency, and poor cost controlling. Practitioners are encouraged to go beyond the introductory information provided here to truly understand the qualities of specific tests used in practice and research.

STATE-OF-THE ART WORK IN OCCUPATIONAL THERAPY

No occupational therapy intervention should be commenced without some form of evaluation to determine the extent of the problem. It is essential to provide ongoing information regarding performance changes as a result of occupational therapy services. This is easier said than done. Few standardized measures exist in occupational therapy that are relevant to the observations needed. Thus, while the profession must support the continued development of standardized instruments that measure occupations, occupational performance, and occupational context interactions, this lack of available instruments for clinical and research purposes cannot be used to avoid the assessment process altogether or as an excuse to arbitrarily develop a site-specific process, neglecting the importance of psychometrics. Even with managed care and the rapidly decreasing length of hospital stays, occupational therapists must introduce evaluation procedures to support intervention planning. Also, communication of reliable, valid test results is essential to avoid unnecessary, costly reevaluation and facilitate transitions and communication between components of the health care system. Transferring meaningful evaluation outcomes between occupational therapy practitioners at different sites or levels of care can increase treatment efficacy and cost efficiency.

Similarly, with the rapid return to home or termination of service occurring in many programs, assessment of abilities may be as important as defining disabilities. Identification of skill strengths and assets that will support return to a specific level of independent living or context can be more critical than identification of ability deficits. Last, the emergence of the occupational therapy practitioner involvement with caregivers require that he or she evaluate this critical component for treatment planning. Assessing caregiver needs and interactions as well as competence and training outcomes is rapidly increasing in clinical importance.

While the Rasch Model is refining our evaluation approach in occupational therapy, we still need to consider further methods to evaluate the impact of the interaction between a person and specific environmental conditions in occupational therapy, as well as the reciprocal communication between individuals such as client-therapist, individual-caregiver, parent-child, and program-service delivery system, to fully evaluate human performance in unique contexts. As these methods emerge, the impact of occupational therapy upon individuals will truly be measured and reported. Ecological assessment will be an interesting area to watch.

TECHNOLOGY AND CHANGING APPROACHES TO EVALUATION

Another significant trend that is inevitable will be the rapid introduction of computers to administer, score, and report evaluation outcomes. An occupational therapist will need not only basic test construction and application information, but also fundamental computer literacy, in order to both administer and track test development. Instead of writing a test company for information or sample packets of its evaluation, a practitioner can now go out on the Internet to a testing company, read about the test, and even view a sample before proceeding to place a purchase order, not to mention scanning available options for testing particular skills or abilities. In addition, computer technology will facilitate integration of information from multiple sources (Anatasi & Urbina, 1997). Individual characteristics and performance abilities that are currently evaluated in isolation will be evaluated simultaneously and finally provide the holistic view of occupational performance desired by our practitioners. Physical abilities, emotions and attitudes, task performance and culture, performance contexts and environments—all essential contributors to understanding and describing an individual's real occupational performance—will be synthesized by computers able to integrate testing information from multiple sources into comprehensive descriptions of complex human behavior.

Summary

From a program planning perspective, evaluation can provide data for outcomes studies to substantiate the benefits received from occupational therapy. Cost effectiveness, intervention efficacy, and consumer satisfaction, including the important aspects of quality of life, can be measured by using standardized tests. Ethical, political, and legal concerns will continue to influence the use of standardized tests and challenge the occupational therapy practitioner to keep abreast of developments related to the use of tests and measurements.

Use of the "best practices" available in assessment and evaluation are *essential*, not optional, in occupational therapy. Therapists must be accountable for their assessment results, as assessment results can not only provide access to necessary services but also can prevent individuals from receiving needed services altogether.

References

American Occupational Therapy Association (1994). Uniform terminology for occupational therapy (3rd ed.). *American Journal of Occupational Therapy, 48,* 1047–1054.

American Occupational Therapy Foundation. (1996). *Priorities and resources for research on occupation and health.* Bethesda, MD: Author.

Anatasi, A., & Urbina, S. (1997). *Psychological Testing* (7th ed.). Upper Saddle River: NJ: Prentice Hall.

Asher, I.E. (1996). *Occupational therapy assessment tools: An annotated index* (2nd ed.). Bethesda, MD: American Occupational Therapy Association.

Ayres, A.J. (1989). *Sensory integration and praxis tests.* Los Angeles: Western Psychological Services.

Behavioral Measurement Database Services. (1994). *Health and psychological instruments* (HaPI), Pittsburgh, PA: Author.

Center for Functional Assessment Research (1993). *Functional Independence Measure* (FIM^{SM}) (Version 4.0) Buffalo, NY: State University of New York at Buffalo.

Cooper, R., & Crist, P.A. (1988). Field test analysis and reliability of the Fieldwork Evaluation for the Occupational Therapist. *Occupational Therapy Journal of Research, 8,* 369–379.

Fisher, A.G. (1992). *Assessment of motor and process skills* (Res. ed. 6.1J). Unpublished test manual, Department of Occupational Therapy, Fort Collins, CO: Colorado State University.

Fisher, A.G. (1995). *Assessment of motor and process skills.* Fort Collins, CO: Three Star Press.

Hemphill, B.J. (1982). *The evaluative process in psychiatric occupational therapy.* Thorofare, NJ: Slack.

Kohlman-Thompson, L. (1992). *Kohlman evaluation of living skills (KELS)* (3rd ed.). Bethesda, MD: American Occupational Therapy Association.

McCowan, R.R., Driscoll, M., & Roop, P. (1992). *Educational psychology*, Needham Heights, MA: Allyn & Bacon.

Nitka, A.J. (1984). Defining criterion-referenced tests. In R.A. Berks (Ed.), *A guide to criterion-referenced test construction* (pp. 8–28). Baltimore: Johns Hopkins University Press.

Park, S., Fisher, A.G., & Velozo, C.A. (1994). Using the Assessment of Motor and Processing Skills to compare occupational performance between clinic and home settings. *American Journal of Occupational Therapy, 48*, 697–709.

6 Non-standardized Assessments

Charlotte Brasic Royeen, PHD, OTR, FAOTA
Jeannette Richards, OTR/L

Overview

This chapter presents an introduction to the innate need to "measure" and the critical issues this need may raise. A brief overview of what constitutes standardized assessment and nonstandardized assessments follows. Nonstandardized assessments are defined and illustrations provided for each type: observation, checklist, interview, and screening. The rationale for use of nonstandardized assessments is delineated. Examples of use of nonstandardized assessment in the occupational therapy literature are provided. A theoretical proposition of the relationship of nonstandardized assessments to occupational therapy practice is posed, followed by case examples illustrating the use of nonstandardized assessments. Consideration of issues of verification and trustworthiness of data obtained from nonstandardized assessments is briefly addressed, followed by additional considerations of other types of nonstandardized assessments. Finally, guidelines for using nonstandardized assessments are presented at the end of the chapter.

Introduction

As human beings we have an innate need to understand and organize our world. We like to sort, categorize, or, in some way, make sense of our world in a manner that can be easily communicated to others, be they members of the tribe, colleagues, or patients' families. One might argue that it is our innate need to make sense of or to "order" the world that has contributed to the development of measurement. Measurement involves assigning numbers to objects, events, or situations, according to some rule (Burns & Grove, 1997; Kaplan, 1964). Indeed, measurement as it is currently being conducted expands beyond this quantitative definition, as typically put forth (Linn & Gronlun, 1995) and includes qualitative methods of the assignment of categories or descriptors instead of numbers (Burns & Grove, 1997). Thus, the notion of just what constitutes "measurement" is undergoing revision, along with the debate over quantitative/qualitative research (Solomon, 1991). Indeed, some have argued for the increased use of ethnographic or qualitative research strategies as a form of measurement in occupational therapy practice (Spencer, Krefting, & Mattingly, 1993).

Measurement, as commonly used, may also be associated with the concept of tests. We are typically socialized to think of quantitative "tests" as the ultimate way to assess people, objects, or things. Indeed, as a society we are, perhaps, a bit too much involved with standardized tests and their outcomes as conveying absolute truth. Consider the following:

1. Did your entrance into occupational therapy school depend, in part, upon SAT or GRE scores?
2. Did passing your driving test really mean you would be a safe, reliable, and courteous driver?
3. Will passing the examination given by National Board for the Certification of Occupational Therapy (NBCOT) mean that you will be a "good" occupational therapy practitioner? Will a higher score mean that you will be a better therapist?

Are any of these statements really true?

Certainly the first one is—that you needed SAT or GRE scores for entry into occupational therapy school. The GRE and the SAT are standardized tests with standardized scores. Did the score you receive really reflect your academic potential and performance? Probably not completely.

Consider the second question—does completion of a standardized driving test evaluation mean you are a good, or even competent, driver? Having recently moved to Nebraska, I had to take a written driving test in a standardized manner, after having successfully driven (with no accidents) on the East Coast for over 20 years. Yet, I flunked my standardized driving examination.

My brother-in-law would say that this was well deserved, but I would argue that my driving is all right.

The third question, concerning passing the national certification examination for occupational therapy, poses another complex dilemma: Just what does passing this standardized test mean in practice?

This brings us to the thorny issue of just what do standardized tests mean?

Simply put, outcomes from standardized tests allow us to consider performance in a restricted area, under prescribed conditions, compared to some reference group of individuals (Cermak, 1989). It means no more, no less. As identified in an earlier chapter, standardized tests have the following characteristics:

- They have been constructed according to prescribed and strict procedures.
- Test items have been selected based upon difficulty and discrimination ability of individual test items.
- Scores are based upon normative or criterion-referenced data.
- The test has described psychometric characteristics of validity and reliability (Royeen, 1992).

Standardized tests are important in almost all aspects of society. Yet, we often take the passing of a standardized test to mean more than it really does. For example, we may confuse competence in driving or in occupational therapy practice with passing of a standardized test of some sort.

It is, therefore, evident that standardized tests in and of themselves cannot measure everything that we may have a need to measure. For this very important reason, another category of measurement tools, nonstandardized assessments, exists.

What Are Nonstandardized Assessments?

In order to most easily understand just what nonstandardized assessment are, let us first look at eight main methods of measurement. They are:

- observation
- interview
- self-report
- scales
- checklists
- protocols
- norm-referenced tests
- criterion-referenced tests.

■ *Table 6.1.* Definitions of Types of Assessment Tools

Type of Tool	Definition
Observation	The process of visually inspecting behavior or other units of study
Interview	The process of inquiry of one person asking another one or more questions
Self-Report	The process of an individual disclosing information about himself in some systematic manner
Scales	The process of rating degree of intensity about a reaction to statements, products, or events
Checklist	The process of documenting the absence or presence of items evaluated using a prescribed listing
Protocol	A prescribed process or procedure for conducting data collection on a unit of interest
Norm-Referenced	A measurement comparing performance of the subject on a test to a comparison group of known characteristics
Criterion-Referenced	A measurement comparing performance of the subject on a test to a pre-established performance level or criterion.

Each of these is defined in Table 6.1.

Table 6.1 presents a beginning level of descriptions and, in certain situations, categories are not mutually exclusive.

Standard III: Screening Standards for Practice for Occupational Therapy (AOTA, 1994, p. 1039) identifies four of these eight methods of measurement as nonstandardized or informal. It is beyond the scope of this introductory textbook to elaborate, but readers should be aware that some types of checklists, observations, interviews, or screening, may indeed be standardized. The specific measurement strategies identified as informal by *AOTA's Standards of Practice* are:

- observations
- checklists
- interviews
- screening.

DESCRIPTION OF NONSTANDARDIZED ASSESSMENTS

To give the reader a good understanding of the four main categories on nonstandardized assessments as identified by AOTA, each will now be explained in more detail, and examples from the occupational therapy literature will be presented.

Observation Defined as a Nonstandardized Assessment

Nonstandardized observation refers to the collection of data through visual inspection of events, environments, or activities, in a manner that is not preordained or prescribed.

Example of observation as a nonstandardized assessment. This is probably the single most prevalent method of evaluation that experienced occupational therapists use. Examples may be when

- you look at posture, symmetry, and fluidity of motion while someone engages in an activity
- you visually inspect a classroom for flow patterns, noise patterns, and visual demands
- you watch an individual who has had a stroke get dressed in his or her home environment
- you observe an individual who has had brain damage figure out how to get from one end of the clinic to the other, navigating around tables, people, and chairs.

For occupational therapists, nonstandardized observations of clients engaged in activities are critically important. Observations of an individual's performance can contribute valuable information to our understanding of an individual's ability to engage successfully in various occupations.

Checklists Defined as a Nonstandardized Assessment

Nonstandardized checklists are those checklists lacking data about how the checklist should be used, normative data on performance of individuals concerning the checklist, and where validity and reliability are unknown.

Example of checklists as a nonstandardized assessment. In occupational therapy, nonstandardized checklists are extremely common. Almost every dressing evaluation involves some sort of nonstandardized checklist. The same may be said of many feeding and bathing assessments. It is simply a method of documenting client performance in some sort of recorded format.

Interview Defined as a Nonstandardized Assessment

A nonstandardized interview is what almost every occupational therapist does with almost every client during the first moments of clinical interaction. The greeting and followup questioning of "How are you doing?" or "Tell me how it has been going" often lead to probes or questions such as, "Can you tell me more about that?" or "And what did you do then?" Such questions reveal much to the therapist about the cognitive, affective, and physical status of the client since their last interaction.

Example of interview as a nonstandardized assessment. Probably one of the most common examples is when the occupational therapist first meets with the client's family members. It is rare that the first meeting consists of a battery of standardized tests. Rather, the occupational therapist usually asks a series of questions, not necessarily prescribed or previously thought out, trying to elicit more information and understanding about the client and his or her occupational patterns and family setting.

Screening Defined as a Nonstandardized Assessment

Screening is a process of quickly discerning salient aspects of potential problems in human performance, as revealed by a short, systematic process of data collection concerning a client, in the absence of standardized procedures or normative data for comparison.

Example of screening as a nonstandardized assessment. In pediatrics, the administration of reflex testing, observations of the child on the playground, and teacher interview might constitute a nonstandardized screening. In adult physical dysfunction, the neurological mental status examination is typically a nonstandardized screening tool for determination of classification (Aminoff, Greenberg, & Simon, 1996).

WHY ARE NONSTANDARDIZED ASSESSMENTS USED?

The rationales for the use of nonstandardized assessments can be many and multifaceted. The main reasons or rationales are summarized in Table 6.2. The table shows that the reason nonstandardized assessments are so common is that they are fast, inexpensive, and easy to use.

Most important, however, is the fact that for most of what we as occupational therapists are interested in, few standardized assessments exist! For example, as occupational therapists we are typically interested in performance components (individual ability), performance areas (activity), and the performance context (environment). Try to think about the standardized tests with which you are familiar and that might be appropriate to assess:

- individual ability or performance components
- activity or performance area
- performance context or environment.

In which area did you identify the most standardized tests? The answer is typically in performance components, that is, a multitude of standardized tests exists for evaluation of performance components or underlying factors related to human function. However, significantly fewer assessments exist for performance areas or environments. If no standardized tests exist, occupational therapists must use nonstandardized assessments for their evaluative process. Simply stated, nonstandardized assessments are used for the measurement of areas not covered by standardized tests.

■ *Table 6.2.* Main Reasons Nonstandardized Assessments Are Used in Occupational Therapy

- Easy to administer
- Extensive training not necessary
- Standardized evaluations often not in existence
- Inexpensive
- Highly portable
- Take little time
- Often performed in context
- Typically noninvasive
- Relatively easy to teach to others for monitoring
- Superficially easy to interpret—long scoring methods not required

Recall that standardized assessments are constructed according to strict procedures, and that test items are selected using statistically based criteria for item analysis and item discrimination, whereas nonstandardized assessments are not. Typically, either the strict procedures for development of the nonstandardized assessment or the statistical data on item analysis, or both, are lacking. As identified by Dunn (1989), the outcome is that one has different types of data resulting from standardized and nonstandardized tests. Standardized tests can produce "objective" data that are quantified and referenced to an acknowledged norm. Nonstandardized tests can produce data that are more "subjective," with unknown relevance to an external group but with great relevance to the individual client.

This issue of relevance and authentic assessment is critical for occupational therapy evaluation. Dunn (1993) identifies it as the consideration of the context, or person-environment fit, as do Letts, Law, Rigby, Cooper, Stewart, & Strong (1994). Nonstandardized assessments lend themselves better to considering these factors in evaluation.

Now, let us see how nonstandardized assessment is represented in selected occupational therapy literature.

REPRESENTATION OF NONSTANDARDIZED ASSESSMENTS IN SELECTED OCCUPATIONAL THERAPY LITERATURE

Observation

In their study of the development of in-hand manipulation and its relationship with activities, Humphrey, Jewell, & Rosenberger (1995) used an observation protocol to measure in-hand manipulation of spoons, buttons, and crayons in children aged 2 through 7. Since there is not yet a standardized test of in-hand manipulation in children, the authors developed a protocol for observation of such tasks. Materials and instructions for the observational protocol were standardized for this study. Though this sounds like a standardized test, it is not, because there are no normative or criterion data provided. The instrument possesses unknown psychometric properties for stability of the assessment over time (reliability) and whether it is actually measuring what it purports to measure (validity).

However, the research investigators did ascertain interrater reliability, that is, they documented that the nonstandardized assessment could be reliably used across therapists. When using nonstandardized assessments, such interrater reliability is critical for both research and the use of the instrument in practice settings.

Checklists

Checklists are very, very common in the practice of occupational therapy. We have checklists for cooking, for dressing, for wheelchair checkout, for toileting and bathing, and for sensory testing, to name just a few. However, most checklists are "home grown" creations of the site or setting, and few make it to publication of any sort.

An exception to this is the *Neurobehavioral Specific Impairment Checklist* (Arnadottir, 1988). It is a comprehensive 10-page checklist concerning neurobehavioral functioning of an adult. A sample is presented in Table 6.3.

Table 6.3 is a rather typical checklist format. As stated by Arnadottir, the checklist is "used for teaching purposes during the therapist's training as a

■ *Table 6.3.* **Sample of Checklist Items from the "Neurobehavioral Specific Impairment Checklist" of Arnadottir (1988)**

Activities of Daily Living (ADL) Functions	Neurobehavioral Impairment Score		
	Present	Absent	Comment
Ideational Apraxia			
1. Does not know what to do with shirt, pants, or socks.	[ ]	[ ]	
2. Misuses clothes. Starts to put leg into armhole or arm into leghole.	[ ]	[ ]	
(a) other apraxia:			
Unilateral Body Neglect			
1. Does not dress the affected body side.	[ ]	[ ]	
2. Does not pull down shirt all the way on the affected side, or shirt gets stuck on the affected shoulder without the person's trying to correct it or realizing what is wrong.	[ ]	[ ]	
Somatoagnoisa			
1. Starts putting legs into armholes or arms into legholes.	[ ]	[ ]	
2. Other body-scheme disorders:			

Arnadottir, G. (1990). *The brain and behavior: Assessing cortical dysfunction through activities of daily living.* St. Louis: Mosby. pp.234–244.

guideline for identifying types of neurobehavioral impairments" (1988, p. 234). The checklist then, is a guide for systematic progression through a series of evaluating steps in the process of problem identification with a client.

Interview

The nonstandardized interview is, perhaps, one of the most exciting and content-rich assessment tools an occupational therapist can use. A study by McComas, Kosseim, and Macintosh (1995) illustrates the nonstandardized interview. In their study of client satisfaction with seating clinic services, four simple questions served as the foundation for hour-long interviews with consumers of services. These questions have been adapted for generic application as presented:

1. What do you think of the seating clinic?
2. How can we make this service better?
3. What is your feeling about the seating inserts you have had to date?
4. Suppose I were a parent with a child requiring seating clinic services. What would you advise me to do? (p. 981).

Since the interview occurred with a focus group format, clients were free to elaborate upon questions, compare answers within the group, and follow through on thoughts and feelings that each question prompted.

Such an approach reflects the flexibility typically seen in qualitative interviewing, which many consider to be synonymous with nonstandardized interview formats.

Screening

The use of nonstandardized screening tools in occupational therapy is prevalent. A screening tool for referral to occupational therapy in home and community health by Johnson (1996) is a most appropriate use of a screening instrument. It is presented in Table 6.4.

Review of Table 6.4 reveals that the nonstandardized screening tool provides the occupational therapist in home and community health a *systemic* way to assist other caregivers in determination of when referral to occupational therapy is appropriate and desirable. Such instrumentation is an efficient method of increasing the cost effectiveness of occupational therapy services, by reducing inappropriate referrals and increasing appropriate referrals.

RELATIONSHIP OF NONSTANDARDIZED ASSESSMENTS TO OCCUPATIONAL THERAPY PRACTICE

Though scant attention is given to it in the literature, more consideration in outcomes research and evidence-based practice should be given to the questions

■ *Table 6.4.* **Screening Tool for Occupational Therapy Referrals by Johnson (1996)**

When evaluating the patient for independence in the following areas, answer the following questions first:

1. Does this person need to be able to do this task?
2. Does this person want to do this task?
3. Is there a reasonable expectation that this person might be able to do this task with appropriate intervention?

Problems noted in any of the following areas constitute criteria for an occupational therapy referral for further evaluation.

Feeding
— Difficulty getting food to mouth
— Inability to feel himself or herself
— Inability to get food on utensil
— Pocketing food
— Coughing after eating or drinking

Mobility
— Activities limited by pulmonary status
— Getting "stuck" in bed
— Inability to transfer in and out of tub and shower
— Difficulty propelling and guiding wheelchair
— Listing to one side while sitting

Perceptual Motor Skills
— Getting "tangled up" in clothing
— Inability to find things in drawers
— Bumping into furniture or doorways
— Cannot complete an activity successfully
— Cannot demonstrate what was just said

Home Safety
— Inability to go out of house in case of emergency
— Difficulty using phone
— Inability to get through doorways or to telephone

Grooming and Hygiene
— Inability to use tub and shower safely
— Difficulty reaching parts of body
— Poor oral hygiene

Toileting
— Unsafe methods of getting on and off toilet
— Unsteady balance on toilet
— Difficulty manipulating undergarments

Dressing
— Difficulty donning shoes and socks
— Problems with manipulation of closures
— Staying in pajamas instead of getting dressed

Upper Extremity Function
— Inability to sign name
— Difficulty manipulating small objects
— Decreased sensation in hands
— Joint deformity
— Limitations in arm movement

Cognitive Skills
— Inability to follow medication dosage schedule
— Difficulty making change or with simple math
— Poor orientation or problem solving

Homemaking
— Inability to prepare simple meals
— Inability to transport food safely
— Inability to recognize unsafe situations

Johnson, K. (1996). Screening tool for occupational therapy referrals. *Home and Community Health Special Interest Section Newsletter, 3 (3)*, 1–2. Used with permission.

"What is best practice?" and "What is bad practice?" In my clinical and continuing education work, I have come to the conclusion that these concepts may be defined, very simply, as follows:

> *Best practice* is solving the right problem *with clients*, i.e., the problem they care about most and that which is most interfering with their occupational performance.

> *Bad practice* is solving the wrong problem *for clients*, i.e., solving a problem that is not relevant to them or which is relatively unimportant to them but highly valued by the therapist.

Why should we consider what is best practice and what is bad practice in a chapter on nonstandardized assessments? Simply stated, nonstandardized assessments can efficiently and effectively assist us to solve the right problem for the individual client, as part of occupational therapy service. The following case scenarios show just some of the ways that nonstandardized assessments can be used to promote "best practice" in occupational therapy.

CASE EXAMPLES ILLUSTRATING BEST PRACTICE IN OCCUPATIONAL THERAPY USING NONSTANDARDIZED ASSESSMENTS

Clinical case examples follow that illustrate how nonstandardized assessments can be effectively used in the practice setting.

Case Example One

Mrs. Andres was making good progress in the rehabilitation process following a cerebral vascular accident. Discharge was planned in 7 days. Her occupational therapist, Lourdes, scheduled a home evaluation to assess her ability to function in her own home environment.

Upon visiting Mrs. Andres's home, Lourdes observed that the front entrance had three steps. As Mrs. Andres was walking up the stairs, Lourdes noticed that she appeared unstable. Lourdes made a note to recommend installation of hand rails on the right side of the entry to coincide with use of Mrs. Andres's unaffected body side.

Inside the house, Lourdes further observed Mrs. Andres in the kitchen as she opened the refrigerator to get a drink, opened the oven door to insert a baking dish, and set the table for dining. Lourdes noted that Mrs. Andres performed these tasks safely, using techniques learned in occupational therapy sessions.

Lourdes continued to observe Mrs. Andres in the bathroom, getting in and out of the tub using a transfer bench, as well as sitting on the toilet. Lourdes also observed Mrs. Andres in her bedroom and living room, as she sat on the furniture in those rooms. Lourdes looked for safety issues such as unsecured rugs, unsteady furniture, and the placement of the telephone, light switches, etc. At the end of the home evaluation, Lourdes took Mrs. Andres back to the rehabilitation unit and discussed safety needs regarding an exterior hand rail. Mrs. Andres concurred. A report for all of the team members was completed, saying that Mrs. Andres was able to perform safely in her home environment, with the exception of the need for hand rails to be installed at the front entry of the house. ∎

In Case Example One, an observational process of looking at the client's home environment was the nonstandardized assessment. A home environment checklist might have been used.

Case Example Two

Anastasia, an occupational therapist, scheduled an interview with Mr. Stone, who had been admitted to the psychiatric unit the previous day, with a diagnosis of situational depression secondary to the loss of his job. Anastasia reviewed his chart, looking at Mr. Stone's history and any recommended precautions.

Anastasia met with Mr. Stone in a quiet area and asked a series of open-ended questions to elicit his story. The questions helped Anastasia learn of Mr. Stone's values, habits, family patterns and support, as well as strengths and areas of concern. She also noted his nonverbal communication such as eye-contact, body posture, use of hands, and head position. She explored occupations, other than work, which Mr. Stone believed were meaningful to him. Anastasia also explored Mr. Stone's ability to follow directions and sequence actions by asking him to help her reorganize the furniture configuration in the room.

With information elicited during this nonstandardized assessment process, Anastasia was able to identify goals for exploration with the client and treatment team. ∎

Case Example Two illustrates the first phase of a functional evaluation in a mental health setting, using nonstandardized assessment procedures including chart review, activity analysis, and interview.

Case Example Three

Mr. Diaz had been admitted to a long-term-care center following a decline in his ability to care for himself in his own home. Darnell, an occupational therapist, was asked to screen him for the possible need for occupational therapy services. Darnell reviewed the chart and then went to Mr. Diaz's room for a screening assessment.

Darnell introduced herself and explained the reason for her visit. She tried to engage Mr. Diaz in social conversation, but Mr. Diaz appeared lethargic and slow to respond. Darnell noticed that his wheelchair was much too large for him and that he was leaning to the right while sitting in the chair. As part of a screening assessment, Darnell asked Mr. Diaz to raise his hands over his head. He was unable to lift them more than 10 inches off of his lap.

Based upon Mr. Diaz's poor sitting posture in the wheelchair, lethargy and poor upper extremity function, Darnell decided to request a referral for an occupational therapy evaluation. She plans to fully evaluate Mr. Diaz's upper extremity function, cognitive status, and abilities, as well as wheelchair specifications and posture while sitting. ∎

Case Example Three illustrates the screening process using nonstandardized assessments, specifically chart review, observation, and informal interview.

Case Example Four

Carmen is a school-based occupational therapist and has been working with Philip, a third grader, for the last 12 weeks—the amount of time her agency has had the contract for provision of occupational therapy services to that particular Local Education Agency (LEA). Carmen "inherited" an Individualized Educational Program (IEP) for Philip that she had to follow. The IEP prescribed a focus on performance components underlying handwriting, i.e., eye-hand coordination training, visual tracking training, and figure-ground discrimination training. Carmen had to document changes in performance levels for these activities. She set up a series of worksheets that require letter tracing, line and shape cutting, and cursive writing of the name Philip.

Carmen will use Philip's performance on the worksheets to monitor progress in performance components for the rest of the school year. ∎

Case Example Four illustrates use of nonstandardized performance measures, in this case worksheets, to assess progress and change during treatment services.

Now that we have a clear understanding of what nonstandardized assessments are and how they are used, we will look at appropriate considerations underlying their use: their verification and trustworthiness.

CONSIDERATION OF VERIFICATION AND TRUSTWORTHINESS OF NONSTANDARDIZED ASSESSMENTS

The minimal standard often set or used for nonstandardized assessments is establishment of interrater reliability. *Interrater reliability* refers to the procedure to document or give assurance that different therapists using the same nonstandardized tool will get the same result. In cases of quantitative nonstandardized assessments, this is very, very important. In cases of qualitative nonstandardized assessments, such as some forms of observations and interview, this is not relevant in the same manner.

Interrater reliability is a specialized form of reliability. Overall, *reliability* refers to the ability of a tool to consistently measure the same thing over time and between raters. Concerning nonstandardized assessment, it addresses the trustworthiness of the data derived from the assessment.

Another consideration is verification. *Verification* of nonstandardized assessments pertains to how one authenticates or verifies the data. You may obtain information from other assessments that confirms your findings, or other team members or the client may confirm or agree with the findings.

Table 6.5 presents a summary overview of strengths and weaknesses related to quantitative psychometric considerations of nonstandardized assessments.

ADDITIONAL CONSIDERATIONS

In this section, four additional types of nonstandardized assessments identified by Fink (1993) will be introduced. These are physical examinations, clinical scenarios, record review, and assessment of performance. Each will be discussed in turn. Remember that categories of nonstandardized assessments are not necessarily mutually exclusive and that there may be some overlap or relationships across categories.

Physical Examination

This refers to a category of nonstandardized assessments typically employed in medicine. This assessment refers to the collection of data directly from

■ *Table 6.5.* Strengths and Weaknesses of Nonstandardized Assessments (in part, adapted from Fink, 1993)

Type of Nonstandardized Assessment	Strengths and Weaknesses
Observation	+ May be only way to look at context and the environment. + Provides actual "slice of life" view of client. + Readily adaptable for home environment assessments, accessibility assessments, etc. + Firsthand or primary information. + Often allows discovery of unanticipated information. − Reliability of observation requires considerable structure in format and training. − Very time consuming. − Can be very expensive. − May be susceptible to the Hawthorn Effect.
Interviews	+ Allows for probes or follow-up of meaning when in person. + Can collect from people who otherwise may not be able to respond (for example, those visually impaired, immobile, etc.) + Commonly used in preliminary research or preliminary clinical interactions. + Allows for in-depth understanding of phenomenon or person. − Time consuming. − Expensive. − May require considerable training. − Unusual responses require high-level interpretation.
Checklists	+ Quick. + Possess great face validity. + Intuitively easy to understand. + Extensive training usually not required. + Portable and inexpensive. − Other types of validity not assured. − Interrater reliability required. − May lack theoretical reference. − May risk "recipe" flavor, lacking individualization.
Screening	+ Can save time. + Can assist in identification of individuals for services who otherwise would not be identified. + Usually very portable. + Usually relatively inexpensive. − Unknown "hits and misses," i.e., correct and not correct identification of problems.

Fink, A. *Evaluation fundamentals: Guiding health programs, research and policy.* Newbury Park, CA: Sage.

visual, tactile, and auditory examination of a patient or client. The simplest example of this may be visual inspection of the ear canal to determine whether there is an inner ear infection. It provides first-hand information but is expensive, labor intensive, and relatively intrusive (Fink, 1993).

Clinical Scenarios

This type of nonstandardized assessment is not yet prevalent in occupational therapy. It can be used to assesses problem solving, judgment, or cognitive ability. It would be used if a client were presented with a scenario and then asked, "What would you do if?" or "What would happen if?" The method is very easy to use to gather information, but it is difficult to assess what is really going on if the subject's responses are way "off the mark."

Record Review

This should be the most common form of nonstandardized assessment there is. It should be, indeed, the first step in the sequence of evaluation and can be part of the screening, in which the occupational therapist reviews all records, materials, and documents pertinent to the client. It is a relatively easy form of information gathering, but the accuracy of the data is unknown and is dependent upon the accuracy of the records presented.

Assessment of Performance

This is often called *authentic assessment* (Linn & Gronlund, 1995) and is what occupational therapists most typically do: observe client performance of a task in the natural environment. It may also be considered to be *criterion referenced,* in that there is typically an outcome performance that the patient or client is trying to achieve and that is to be rated by the occupational therapist. It involves doing something and not just knowing about it. Furthermore, it involves consideration of the process as well as the product of the activity being performed (Linn & Gronlund, 1995). It is what we as occupational therapists, in theory, lay claim to, but we have published relatively little about it, in terms of assessments.

Goal Attainment Scaling

This is another type of nonstandardized assessment that is individualized to the client. There are eight steps in goal attainment scaling:

1) Identify the goal.
2) Identify specific processes to be addressed.
3) Identify what events or behaviors are desired outcomes.
4) Identify the method of data collection to monitor targeted outcome behaviors.

5) Establish expected or desired level of performance or outcome behavior.

6) Identify worst-case outcome, best-case outcome, and in-between level of outcome.

7) Identify areas of overlap between best- and worst-case outcomes.

8) Identify client performance (Ottenbacher & Cusik, 1993; Royeen, 1993).

Portfolio Assessment

This is a relatively new area of nonstandardized assessment that consists of a collection of projects, outcomes, or other tangible products of the efforts put forth by a client in a particular area. These are comprehensive assessment tools, which are time-consuming to compile and coordinate.

Projection Techniques

This is probably one of the oldest nonstandardized assessments employed by occupational therapists. Typically, it has been used in psychosocial occupational therapy, in art activities wherein the client is asked to describe or "project" what they see, perceive, or feel about something in a media representation. Projection techniques have great power in revealing underlying psychological processes, but they are also labor intensive and subject to wide variation in interpretation.

Given this overview of the majority of classifications of nonstandardized assessments, the next section of this chapter will present guidelines for using these assessments in occupational therapy practice.

GUIDELINES FOR USING NONSTANDARDIZED ASSESSMENTS

The appropriate and effective use of nonstandardized assessments requires the occupational therapist to have a solid theoretical basis and sound clinical reasoning. To that end, the following simple guidelines should be followed when employing nonstandardized assessments (adapted from Linn & Gronlund, 1995).

1) First, the nonstandardized assessment should be selected based upon its relevance to the domain to be measured (performance components, performance area or role performance or occupational performance).

2) Second, a comprehensive evaluation requires use of more than one single assessment. A comprehensive evaluation should include a variety of procedures and methods as well as types of data collection.

3) Third, assessment is always a means to an end and never an end in itself. One should, therefore, always be sensitive to client cues and never overly stress or fatigue the client.

Two additional issues are brought forth for consideration. One is use of a client-centered approach, in which the occupational therapist works in collaboration with the client so that it is the client's concerns that are addressed (Pollock, 1993).

The second issue pertains to cultural sensitivity. Research demonstrates variation in response style and performance motivation between Caucasians and African Americans (Evans & Salim, 1992). In all likelihood, other variations exist for other racial or cultural groups. Therefore, use of nonstandardized assessments should always allow for cultural variation.

Summary

Evaluation represents a large part of the work that occupational therapists perform. They depend on the results of assessment tools to guide client treatment and the discharge plan. Standardized assessments are limited in number and must be used within the restricted and prescribed conditions of the reference group, which often imposes artificial conditions. This chapter discussed use of nonstandardized assessments in occupational therapy practice. Particularly, such tools are used to establish baseline performance of strengths and limitations in the best practice concept of solving the right problems for the client. Nonstandardized assessments should be chosen carefully, considering strengths and limitations of the instrument and following the guidelines discussed in this chapter.

References

Alston, R.J., & McCowan, C.J. (1994). Aptitude assessment and African American clients. The interplay between culture and psychometrics in rehabilitation. *Journal of Rehabilitation, I*, 41–46.

Aminoff, M.J., Greenberg, D.A., Simon, R.P. (1996). *Clinical neurology* (3rd ed.). Stamford, CT: Appleton & Lange.

Arnadottir, G. (1990). *The brain and behavior: Assessing cortical dysfunction through activities of daily living.* St. Louis: Mosby.

American Occupational Therapy Association. (1994). Standards of practice for occupational therapy. *American Journal of Occupational Therapy, 48,* 1039–1043.

Burns, N., & Grove, S.K. (1997). *The practice of nursing research: Conduct, critique, and utilization* (3rd ed.). Philadelphia: Saunders.

Cermak, S. (1989). Norms and scores. *Physical and Occupational Therapy in Pediatrics, 9* (1), 91–123.

Dunn, W. (1989). Validity. *Physical and Occupational Therapy in Pediatrics, 9* (1), 149–169.

Dunn, W. (1993). Measurement of function: Actions for the future. *American Journal of Occupational Therapy, 47*, 357–359.

Evans, J., & Salim, A.A. (1992). A cross cultural test of the validity of occupational therapy assessment with patients with schizophrenia. *American Journal of Occupational Therapy, 46*, 8, 685–695.

Fink, A. (1993). *Evaluation fundamentals: Guiding health programs, research and policy.* Newbury Park, CA: Sage.

Goodman, S.H., Sewell, D.R., Cooley, E.L., & Leavitt, N. (1994). Assessing level of adaptive functioning: The role functioning scale. *Community Mental Health, 29*, 119–131.

Johnson, K. (1996). Screening tool for occupational therapy referrals. *Home and Community Special Interest Section Newsletter 3*, 1.

Humphrey, R., Jewell, K., & Rosenberger, R.C. (1995). Development of in-hand manipulation and relationship with activities. *American Journal of Occupational Therapy, 49*, 763–771.

Kaplan, A. (1964). *The conduct of inquiry: Methodology for behavioral science.* New York: Chandler.

Letts, L., Law, M., Rigny, P., Cooper, B., Stewart, D., & Strong, S. (1994). Person-environment assessments in occupational therapy. *American Journal of Occupational Therapy, 48*, 608–618.

Linn, R.L., & Gronlund, N.E. (1995). *Measurement and assessment in teaching.* Englewood Cliffs, NJ: Simon and Schuster.

McComas, J., Kosseim, M., & Macintosh, D. (1995). Client-centered approach to develop a seating clinic satisfaction questionnaire: A qualitative study. *American Journal of Occupational Therapy, 49*, 980–993.

Ottenbacher, K.J., & Cusik, A. (1993). Discriminative versus evaluative assessment: Some observations on goal attainment scaling. *American Journal of Occupational Therapy, 47*, 249–354.

Pollack, N. (1993). Client-centered assessment. *American Journal of Occupational Therapy, 47*, 298–301.

Royeen, C.B. (1992). Educationally related assessment. In C.B. Royeen (Ed.), *AOTA's self study series: Classroom applications for school based practice.* Bethesda, MD: American Occupational Therapy Association.

Royeen, C.B. (1997). Measurement. In C.B. Royeen (Ed.), *The research primer.* Bethesda, MD: American Occupational Therapy Association.

Solomon, G. (1991). Transcending the qualitative-quantitative debate: The analytic and systemic approaches to educational research. *Educational Researcher, 20*, 10–18.

Spencer, J., Krefting, L., & Mattingly, C. (1993). Incorporation of ethnographic methods in occupational therapy assessment. *American Journal of Occupational Therapy, 47*, 303–309.

7 Assessment Selection

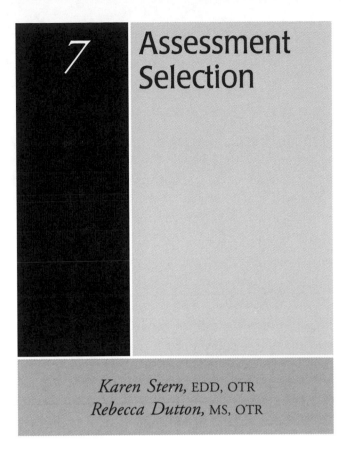

Karen Stern, EDD, OTR
Rebecca Dutton, MS, OTR

Overview

An integral aspect of the evaluation process is the selection of the most appropriate assessments to evaluate an individual's current level of functioning. Later, assessments are chosen to determine whether the individual has made progress during the intervention process. Assessment selection is affected by a variety of factors, such as expressed client needs, frame of reference, context of intervention, and phases of evaluation. This chapter will describe the assessment selection process. The overall process of tool selection will be illustrated through the presentation of case examples.

Introduction

Assessment selection refers to the process of identifying which tools will provide information essential for determining intervention strategies and courses of action. It is a complex process that relies on the clinical reasoning skills of the therapist. The therapist considers a number of factors when determining which assessments are appropriate. These include the individual's needs and concerns, the selection of frames of reference, the system in which the therapist works, the various contexts of intervention, and the phases of evaluation. The impact of each of these factors on the selection of appropriate assessments will be explored.

The Individual's Needs and Concerns

When considering which tools to use during an evaluation, the therapist must be aware of the needs and concerns of the individual. Client-centered care ensures that services are relevant to the individual and not just based on a diagnostic category, needs of the institution, or bias of the therapist.

Client needs and concerns require the therapist to use an unstructured interview to get to know the individual. The types of questions asked might include, but not be limited to:

- Which areas are of concern to the individual and family?
- What are the individual's valued and preferred roles, habits, and skills?
- Does the individual want to return to work?
- Did he or she ever help with the housework?
- Does a family member want to assume responsibility for assisting the individual with self–care activities?

These questions will provide the therapist with a more comprehensive understanding of the client. Armed with this knowledge, the therapist can then look into his or her battery of tests and assessments.

For example, John has a long history of alcohol abuse and depression and has entered a 28-day inpatient drug and alcohol abuse rehabilitation program. During the initial interview with the occupational therapist, he expressed concerns about how he will manage his time upon discharge, as his activities revolved mainly around drinking. To assist the therapist in determining how John spent his time in the past and how he would like to spend his time in the future, an activity configuration such as the Barth Time Construction (1985) could be administered. This information will provide a starting point for discussing how he organized his time in the past and what changes John would like to make. Other tools, such as the NPI Interest Checklist (Matsutsuyu, 1969), might then be used to determine new areas of interest that might be developed to take the place of previous nonconstructive activities.

It is often difficult to learn the client's true concerns at the beginning of intervention. Some clients and caregivers do not identify their concerns on the first day. For example, clients who are in acute phases of illness may have global concerns, such as "to get well" or "to go home." Clients and caregivers who have never received therapy or been involved in the therapeutic process may not be able to state specific concerns. A parent may be concerned about her son's ability to feed himself but may initially be reluctant to share this thought. Any therapist who has seen a mother's face when her son feeds himself ice cream at his birthday party knows that this is not a trivial concern, but clients and caregivers often feel shy at first about expressing these nonmedical concerns. Even clients and caregivers who have been dealing with a chronic condition may wait a few days before sharing intimate concerns such as "being able to hold my grandchild in my lap," especially if they have been rebuffed in the past by comments from therapists such as "that is not my role." Learning about the client is an ongoing process. As rapport is established during the evaluation process, the client or caregiver should be encouraged to express his or her concerns.

Once the client's concerns are known, the therapist can select tools specific to the area of concern of the client. In the case of the parent concerned about her son's ability to feed himself, an assessment of feeding skills can be made. Another example of how client/caregiver concerns affect assessment selection is the case of Susan. She had a stroke 2 weeks ago and is frustrated about being dependent on the nurses every time she wants a tissue from the nightstand. The therapist should assess what underlying performance components are interfering with the client's ability to perform this and other valued activities within this setting. Thus, the therapist will select procedures that will evaluate specific performance components such as range of motion, muscle strength against gravity, rolling with neck righting, or a strong retraction of the arm.

In addition to understanding the concerns of the individual, the occupational therapist should also talk directly to family members and significant others, because clients and their families often have very different perceptions of what each expects of the other. A client may say that her spouse will do everything for her, but the spouse may not actually be willing or able to do everything. The therapist should assess at least some of the performance areas that are reasonable for the family to expect the client to perform at home, as well as the client's performance components that support independence. For example, a client may be expected to independently get her lunch from the refrigerator but may not be expected to help prepare it.

Addressing client and caregiver concerns taps into intrinsic motivation, encourages the individual to actively participate in the decision-making process, and can create a powerful success experience that strongly influences how this person's life will turn out.

Context

There are many different aspects of context. Several of them will be discussed here, as they affect tool selection. Specifically, this section will address the system, the environmental context, and the temporal context.

THE SYSTEM

The nature of the system in which the occupational therapist practices influences the choice of assessments. Length of stay, types of reimbursement, role delineations, and resources available all affect the evaluation and intervention process.

Length of stay determines the amount of time the therapist has available for the evaluation and intervention process. This is driven in large part by the type of reimbursement for services (for example, Health Maintenance Organization, Private Health Care Insurance, Preferred Provider Plans, Boards of Education, Early Intervention Programs). When the length of stay in a facility is limited (3–4 days, six half-hour treatment sessions, etc.), the evaluation process must proceed quickly. Similarly, if the length of time for evaluation is limited by legislation, such as in a school system or early intervention program, the evaluation must be done in an expeditious manner. This may mean that an evaluation is limited to initial screening tools, followed by limited specific assessments. In an acute inpatient psychiatric unit, assessments such as the Comprehensive Occupational Therapy Evaluation (Brayman & Kirby, 1982) may be used to quickly identify the client's areas of concern. Comprehensive assessment of all areas of concern is impractical in such a situation, as there is insufficient time to assess and provide intervention within the allotted time. Therefore, the therapist has to be both focused on the areas to be assessed and skilled enough to choose and administer specific assessments. Alternatively, when length of stay is extended, such as in a long-term day program, there may be sufficient time for a more comprehensive evaluation such as the Bay Area Functional Performance Evaluation (BAFPE) (Williams & Bloomer, 1987) to determine cognitive and psychosocial components.

With increased emphasis on accountability by those who pay for services, the cost of the evaluation and intervention process must be justified. This requires the therapist to limit the selection of assessments to those that address the immediate needs of the client, given the context. Though the choice of the assessment tool should be left up to the therapist, some third party payers specify the types of assessments they will agree to cover. However, ethically it is incumbent on the therapist to be sure that the assessment meets the needs of the client.

The roles and responsibilities in the practice setting affect the practice of occupational therapy within that setting. There is overlap among the practice of the various professionals in any setting. Each facility specifies the roles and responsibilities for each member of the team. For example, in some short-term inpatient psychiatric units, nursing staff are responsible for assessment and intervention of self-care activities. Thus, the occupational therapist would not replicate services by assessing the individual's performance in self-care activities, but might assess specific areas as indicated by the reports of other professionals. In some rehabilitation settings, the occupational therapist may assess transfers and cognition, while in other settings transfers may be shared with the physical therapist, while cognition is shared with the neuropsychologist. In a school setting, the occupational therapist must focus on areas relevant to the educational needs of the child, which may include handwriting but in some settings would not include dressing skills.

Some institutions specify the type of assessments used by the team. For example, different sections of the Functional Independence Measure (FIM) (Jette, Davis, Cleary, et al., 1986) may be assigned to specific team members, such as dressing for the occupational therapist and incontinence for the nurse. Each team member contributes his or her scores to produce a single composite score for the client. This composite score must be agreed upon by the entire team for every client admitted to that particular unit. Similarly, in a multidisciplinary early intervention program, one team member might administer the Denver II Developmental Screening Test (Frankenberg, Dodds, Archer, et al., 1991) to every child, while the rest of the team observes.

The resources of the facility also affect the type of assessments available. If there is a limited amount of space in the assessment or intervention area, or if many members of the team share space, assessments that require much space or permanent structures will not be feasible. If there are a limited number of clients who need a particular type of assessment such as work hardening, the therapist may not be able to justify the cost of expensive assessment materials. One such assessment, the *Valpar Components Work Samples* (Valpar International Corporation, 1986) costs from $1,000 to $4,000 per subtest. A less expensive assessment that provides similar data may have to be selected, or the therapist may have to refer the client to another facility. On the other hand, in home health care, where the assessment takes place in a natural setting, the tools of everyday life are readily available and can be used in assessment. For example, the therapist can assess safety issues in the client's kitchen, instead of setting up simulated situations in the clinic kitchen.

ENVIRONMENT

The second contextual factor that influences assessment selection is the physical, social, and cultural environment of the individual (AOTA, 1994). In order to select a specific assessment, the therapist must know about the expectations, constraints, and assets of the client's current and/or expected environment. Kielhofner (1985) refers to constraints and expectations as *environmental press*. Practitioners often refer to assets in the environmental context as *environmental resources*.

Environmental press from the social and cultural context may come from the expectations of intervention, the family, and the employer or teachers. For example, in an acute care setting, environmental press may come from the expected environment of the client, such as a subacute rehabilitation program. Two expectations of subacute programs include the amount of therapy time the client will be able to tolerate each day, and whether treatment takes place in a common treatment area where street clothes are required. These two expectations will drive assessment selection and would lead the therapist to select a clinical observation procedure for endurance and dressing skills to determine if the patient is ready for the demands of the new therapy program.

When the client is going to be sent home, it is important to assess the environmental press that comes from expectations of the family. The occupational therapist should talk directly to the family. Does the family expect the client to independently answer the telephone or continue to pay the bills? By listening to the tone of the conversation and watching nonverbal communication, the therapist gets a sense of whether the family is willing to make changes. If the concern expressed by the client and family is for him or her to continue to pay the bills and answer the phone, the therapist may select the Kohlman Evaluation of Living Skills (1992) to assess these areas.

Finally, when the client is ready to return to work or school, the environmental press that is based on the expectations of employers or teachers may need to be assessed. These expectations can be evaluated by talking to employers or teachers and/or by making a site visit. The occupational therapist should explore expectations such as doing classwork without supervision in a noisy classroom or filling out complex forms by writing on small lines at work. These expectations would require tools that assess performance components such as attention span, self-monitoring, and eye-hand coordination, as well as performance areas such as writing.

In addition to environmental press, the occupational therapist should also explore environmental resources when talking to family, teachers, and employers. This includes the culture of the individual. For example, one client lived in a closely knit community and relatives lived only two doors away, so friends and family did all her cooking and cleaning (Levine, 1988). Therefore, a homemaking evaluation would not be needed. Cohen (1988) encourages therapists to look positively at reciprocity, rather than see it as a loss of independence. Similarly, in some cultures homemaking is limited to females, and therefore homemaking skills do not necessarily have to be evaluated for males within that culture. If we are honest with ourselves, we must admit that we all receive assistance for some tasks that we could perform in our daily lives but choose not to do ourselves. Therefore, there may be areas for each client that do not require assessment.

Therapists should seek out information from significant others. A close-knit family may not appreciate the therapist's suggestions, because family members may demonstrate their love for a stricken family member by doing things for him or her. As long as there is consensus among family members and those important to the individual about what the client is expected to do, the therapist should not impose his or her personal values about independence. Of course, if we neglect to ask about environmental press and resources, it is easy to force our values on clients. That is why it is important to talk to significant others in a client's environment and identify performance areas that are "not applicable" before assessment begins. Unfortunately, assessment forms do not prompt therapists to engage in this dialogue, so the therapist has to take the initiative to collect data about environmental press and resources, while engaged in the overall evaluation process.

Environmental press may come from the physical context in the form of architectural barriers or limited physical resources. Before assessing performance areas, the therapist needs to know whether the physical environment will compound or alleviate the client's impairments. The therapist needs to know about barriers such as steps up to the front door, lack of first floor bathrooms and bedrooms, and tightly congested classrooms. A family member is a good source of this type of information about the home environment. A client may be returning to a boarding home with limited cooking facilities.

The occupational therapist may also interview the family to explore environmental resources that are available to support the client. This includes physical as well as financial resources available to the family. Before assessing whether a client can safely transfer onto a tub bench or manage a computerized environmental control unit to turn on lights and answer the telephone, it is important to know whether there is space available for such equipment, as well as funding for it. This information may appear to be a social worker's responsibility, but therapists cannot justify charging clients for assessments that will produce solutions for the physical environment that cannot be implemented.

As you can see, assessment selection is strongly influenced by the expectations, constraints, and assets of the client's physical, social, and cultural environment. Examples of several assessments were provided, but the wide variability of environments would require an exhaustive list. Environmental context introduces considerations that should be considered early in the evaluation process. It has an impact by indicating assessments that would be most important, as well as those that are not necessary.

TEMPORAL CONTEXT

The third contextual factor that influences assessment selection is temporal. Temporal context includes the temporal aspects of the disability status, chronological and developmental age, and the life cycle (AOTA, 1994).

Examining the temporal context of disability status provides critical information about the potential impact of the disability. Clients who are acutely ill have different concerns than those who have already returned to work. Each stage of an illness has a specific pathophysiology that may contribute to the disability. For example, a burn patient may have sensory concerns in the acute stage due to pain but sensory concerns in the postgrafting stage due to a lack of tactile discrimination. One stage requires assessment of a pain baseline, while the later stage requires tests of tactile discrimination, such as two-point discrimination.

Temporal context influences assessment selection. Kaya was a 4-year-old with several developmental delays, including the inability to draw. The reason he was unable to draw changed as the temporal context of his disability changed. Initially, he had difficulties with this task because of severe scapular winging and trunk flexion while sitting unsupported. Two months later, he sat fully erect and had no scapular winging. Yet he still did not draw well, because he could not move his wrist from side to side or supinate his forearm to create a clear line of sight between his eyes and the tip of the crayon. Initially, assessment focused on clinical observation of scapular winging and trunk extension; later assessment focused on clinical observation for dissociated movements of the wrist and forearm. Thus, the choice of which clinical observations to focus on is influenced by the child's stage of development.

Safety is always the first concern when deciding what should be evaluated. For example, when evaluating a client who is sitting up in bed and is acutely ill, it is vital to assess sitting and orthostatic hypotension. The therapist should assess the individual's trunk stability and his or her tendency to faint, before turning away to get clothing during a dressing assessment. Conversely, safety issues may force the therapist not to assess a particular concern. While an occupational therapist would be concerned about a client's ability to return to work, recent hand surgery would contraindicate assessment of finger range of motion, grip strength, and manual dexterity.

Finally, the temporal context includes considering chronological and developmental age. Some tests were developed for specific age groups. Pediatric tests in particular have specified age ranges, such as the Denver II Developmental Screening Test, which is designed for children ages 0 to 6 years. As noted in Chapter 5, which described the importance of psychometric measures for guiding test selection, the therapist must take into consideration the age for which the test was designed. If a test is administered to a client who falls outside the normative age group, standardized scores cannot be used.

Thus, assessment selection is strongly influenced by temporal contexts such as the stage of the disability status, the life cycle, and developmental and chronological age. While a reliable standardized test may provide important information, that information may not be truly helpful to the therapist if it does not accommodate concerns imposed by temporal contexts.

Frames of Reference

The fourth factor that influences assessment selection is frames of reference. The frame of reference provides guidance in the selection of assessment tools and the subsequent interpretation of data collection. "Gathering and reasoning with data is a theoretically informed process that occurs within a framework provided by the model(s) of practice a therapist is using" (Kielhofner, 1996, p. 189). Thus, it is important to select particular assessments that are consistent with the frame of reference.

Each frame of reference delineates the areas of occupational therapy's domain of concern that will be addressed by the occupational therapist. One frame of reference rarely addresses the total domain of concern of occupational therapy. Instead, each tends to focus on particular areas, as it is unrealistic for therapists to evaluate the total domain of concern with every client.

Many factors influence the choice of a frame of reference. Frames of reference may be chosen because of the specific needs of the client or they may be chosen because of factors external to the client, which include the therapist's skills and experience and institutional factors, such as the length of stay and physical resources of the facility. Furthermore, the outcomes desired by the client, his or her family, and the therapist all affect the choice of a frame of reference.

In selecting a frame of reference, several concerns should be addressed. Does the frame of reference address the areas of concern for the individual and/or family members? If the client's concern is how he will structure his time appropriately in the future, the frame of reference selected must include time management in its domain of concern. Does the therapist have an understanding of and expertise with this frame of reference? Does he or she feel comfortable with the implementation of the frame of reference? For example, the use of Allen's Cognitive Disability model is appropriate for individuals with cognitive deficits; however, the therapist must have a thorough understanding of the cognitive levels, the assessment of cognitive levels, and the indepth task analysis required for intervention. While it may be an appropriate choice, if the therapist is not comfortable or experienced in the application of the frame of reference, another frame of reference that addresses this area of function may be more appropriate.

Is the frame of reference appropriate for the length of stay in a particular setting? For example, if an individual will only remain hospitalized for 3 to 4 days, frames of reference that require significant amounts of time to implement will not be useful. A client has significant psychosocial issues that can be addressed by a psychoanalytic frame of reference. However, since this intervention process demands an extended period of time, it would not be an appropriate choice to use in a short-term setting. Once the frame of reference is chosen, it will guide in tool selection. While the frame of reference may not list specific tools to use, it will give guidelines as to the particular areas that need to be evaluated. Some assessment tools are designed specifically for a given frame of reference. For example, if the therapist is using Allen's Cognitive Disability frame of reference, then the Allen Cognitive Level test (Allen, 1990) would be used to determine the cognitive level of the individual. When using a sensory integrative frame of reference, one might use the Sensory Integration and Praxis Tests (Ayres, 1989).

Other assessments may be compatible with several frames of reference. One might use a variety of clinical observations and tests such as the Bruininks-Oseretsky Test of Motor Proficiency (Bruininks, 1978) combined with anecdotal reports from the classroom teacher for information related to motor performance and sensory integrative abilities. Some assessments, particularly assessments of activities of daily living such as the Milwaukee Evaluation of Daily Living Skills (Leonardelli, 1988), are designed to assess a particular performance area without specifying a frame of reference.

It is important to keep in mind that no single frame of reference addresses all the concerns of a particular client. Frames of reference generally address only a limited range of concerns. When allowing a single frame of reference to guide assessment selection, therapists must always be aware that they may have put on blinders that will cause them to ignore many valid concerns. Therapists can avoid this danger by combining frames of reference to produce an unique mix for each client. For example, for a client who has had a stroke, a therapist might use the biomechanical frame of reference to select tests, such as volumetry for edema of the hand and clinical observation for shoulder subluxation, and the neurodevelopmental frame of reference to select tools, such as clinical observation for abnormal muscle tone and impaired automatic reactions. Together, these two frames of reference can provide a comprehensive assessment of the individual.

Frames of reference influence test selection in many ways. The specific concerns of the client prompt the therapist to think about the appropriate frame of reference. The frame of reference then suggests particular assessments to be used. Before proceeding, the therapist must feel comfortable with the frame of reference and have expertise in administering the assessments suggested by that frame of reference. Finally, the therapist must reflect on whether the chosen frame of reference and its assessments will comprehensively meet the individual's needs and be compatible with the setting in which the client is receiving intervention.

Phases of Evaluation

In order to more clearly discusses tool selection, it is helpful to define the various segments of the evaluation process. The first segment is screening, to obtain an overview of the client and his or her potential need for intervention. Following a chart review, an initial half-hour evaluation may include the use of a screening tool, along with clinical observations. This initial phase of evaluation guides subsequent tool selection. The next phase of evaluation involves the use of comprehensive tests which gives a more in-depth picture of the client's abilities. Specialty tests, the next phase of evaluation, are used to give an indepth understanding of one particular area of the client's abilities. During the course of intervention, the therapist makes ongoing observations to determine changes in the client and the need for changes in the intervention plan. These ongoing observations are the final phase of evaluation. Specific examples of assessments that are used at different phases of evaluation and the relationship to frames of reference are listed in Table 7.1. This table is not meant to be an exhaustive list of tests, but it illustrates how frames of reference may guide the choice of assessment and the tools that the therapist may use to collect data at the various phases.

The purpose of standardized screening tests is to quickly detect areas of strengths and concerns and to guide test selection. The purpose of comprehensive tests is to:

- Identify deficits and strengths in performance components that may effect performance areas
- Identify assets and deficits in performance areas
- Provide a baseline for intervention planning
- Provide a detailed baseline to permit documentation of changes in short periods of time.

The purpose of specialty tests is to:

- Supplement comprehensive tests that may add in-depth information about specific areas of concern
- Further assess deficits in performance components and in performance areas
- Confirm specific deficits and strengths in performance areas.

The purpose of ongoing observation is to:

- Identify unanticipated areas of concern
- Supplement comprehensive test data (Dutton, 1995).

The phases of evaluation serve as a guide to assessment selection in conjunction with the needs of the client, the frame of reference, and context of

■ *Table 7.1.* **Examples of Phases of Assessments Specific to Selected Frames of Reference**

Frame of Reference	One Area of Concern	Screening Procedure	Comprehensive Test	Specialty Test	Ongoing Observation
Biomechanical	Range of motion	Observe and estimate range of motion	Formal goniometry	Volumetry	Observe AROM during ADLs
Neuro-developmental treatment	Axial control	Observe ability to sit symmetrically	Axial muscle tone assessment (Dutton, 1997)	None	Handling during transfers
Sensory-motor	Somato–sensory discrimination	Test for stereognosis	Test for somatosensory abilities	Moberg Pick-up Test (Dellon, 1988)	Spontaneous limb use during ADLs
Transfer of training	Perceptual processing (adult)	Screening for visual acuity	Lowenstein O.T. Cognitive Assessment (1990)	Test of Visual–Motor Skills (Gardner, 1986)	Observe for visual neglect during ADLs
Model of human occupation	Values	Interview client about his/her values	Occupational History (Kielhofner, 1995)	Volitional questionnaire	Values patient expresses during ADLs
Acquisitional–activity of daily living	Activities of daily living	Interview client about self-care routines	Kohlman Evaluation of Daily Living Skills (Kohlman–Thompson, 1992)	None	Observe a specific ADL
Acquisitional–play	Play	Family Observation Guide (Hinojosa & Kramer, 1997)	Play History (Takata, 1974)	Test of Playfulness (Bundy, 1997)	Observation of involvement in leisure activities
Sensory integration	Praxis	Quick Neurological Screening Test (Mutti, Sterling & Spalding, 1978)	Bruininks–Oseretsky Test of Motor Proficiency (1978)	Sensory Integration and Praxis Tests (Ayres, 1989)	Ayres clinical observations (Ayres, 1976)
Developmental 0–3 years	Gross coordination	Hawaii Early Learning Profile (HELP) (Furuno, O'Reilly, Hosaka, et al., 1984)	Toddler & Infant Motor Evaluation (TIME) (Miller, 1993)	Alberta Infant Motor Scales (AIMS) (Piper & Darrah, 1994)	Observe gross motor play

intervention. For example, if dysfunction in the area of cognitive components is suspected, an acquisitional frame of reference may be selected to guide the evaluation and intervention process. The therapist may choose to use the *Comprehensive Occupational Therapy Evaluation Scale* (Brayman & Kirby, 1982) as a formal screening tool. If limitations in the area of cognitive components are identified as in need of more indepth assessment, a comprehensive tool such as the Bay Area Functional Performance Evaluation (Williams & Bloomer, 1987) can be administered.

Case Example 1

LATISHA

Latisha is a 28-year-old single female who was diagnosed with schizophrenia, chronic type, 10 years ago. Since that time, she has had multiple admissions to the state psychiatric hospital, the most recent beginning 3 months ago. She is unable to return home to live with her parents, as they are both chronically ill. Latisha does not have the skills to live independently in the community. The plan, with Latisha's consent, is to discharge her to a group home. In order to prepare her for this new living environment, she has been transferred to the transitional living program at the state hospital. The average length of stay in this program is 2 to 3 months.

The assessment selected by the therapist was the Milwaukee Evaluation of Daily Living Skills (MEDLS) (Leonardelli, 1988). What was the rationale for assessment selection? In this setting, the role of the occupational therapist includes responsibility for activities of daily living assessment and intervention. This is consistent with Latisha's needs to be independent in her activities of daily living in the group home. There is adequate time available for comprehensive assessment and intervention. Given Latisha's need to learn new skills, the acquisitional frame of reference was selected. The MEDLS is consistent with the selected frame of reference and was designed specifically for the chronic adult client. There is a good fit between the needs of the individual, the frame of reference, the context in which the evaluation will be performed, and the context to which the client will be going. The MEDLS can also be repeated following intervention, to document functional outcomes. The MEDLS does not require extensive or expensive materials, a critical factor in terms of state institution budgets.

The MEDLS includes both screening and comprehensive evaluation. Based on information from the screening process, Latisha's needs, and the skills required for successful transition to living in the group home, the therapist selected the areas of daily living skills in need of further assessment. The assessment took place in the transitional living unit, which simulates the environment found in many group homes. This is critical, as the assessment data are most accurate when gathered in the client's natural environment. ∎

Case Example 2

RONALD

Ronald is a 69-year-old male who had a right cerebral vascular accident (CVA) 3 weeks ago. Length of stay is expected to be 3 weeks. The first step in the evaluation process is to check his chart for other medical conditions. The CVA is the reason for his current admission, but what other medical conditions might require the therapist to follow precautions? A review of the chart showed that Ronald had a foley catheter, but the diabetes and hypertension that commonly precede a CVA were absent.

The second step is to assess environmental press by reading the chart and talking to Ronald and his wife. Ronald will be discharged to live at home with his wife in a two-story home. The house has six steps with no handrail for the front door and one bathroom on the second floor. Ronald is retired and both he and his wife enjoy volunteering at their local church. His wife does most of the housework, but Ronald enjoys yard work, including gardening and mowing the lawn on his riding mower.

The third step is to assess performance areas, such as independence in self-care. Ronald requires minimal physical assistance for self-care, except for moderate physical assistance for fastenings and cutting food. He ambulates independently with a quad cane.

The fourth step is to let frames of reference guide a thorough and systematic evaluation to determine what underlying deficits are causing his dysfunction in self-care. Individuals with CVAs often have shoulder subluxation, low endurance, edema, and loss of range of motion (ROM). These concerns suggest using the biomechanical frame of reference. The therapist uses clinical observation to quickly determine that Ronald does not have a subluxed shoulder. He does have low endurance, as seen by need for rest during the self-care assessment, and a visibly swollen hand. Volumetry for the swollen hand and an endurance baseline using duration and number of rests required could be done during upcoming assessments. By quickly observing passive ROM, the therapist determines that he does not have any joint contractures of the hemiplegic arm and leg, so a goniometric assessment of ROM is not necessary.

Individuals with CVAs often have abnormal muscle tone and pathological limb synergies, which suggests using the neurodevelopmental (NDT) frame of reference. Dutton (1995) suggests using a decision tree process that takes the individual's temporal context into account. The therapist can begin with the Brunnstrom (1970) assessment of limb synergies, which quickly tells the therapist what stage of recovery the client is in and whether high-level motor tests are appropriate. Ronald has a full upper extremity flexor synergy and moderate to severe spasticity of his arm, so fine motor tests are contraindicated. He has moderate spasticity of his trunk and sits asymmetrically, so high-level tests of automatic reactions, such as equilibrium, are contraindicated. Synergies do not affect Ronald during lower extremity self-care, so further NDT assessment of the lower extremity is not needed.

As part of the ongoing evaluation process, the therapist is able to use clinical observations to screen for perceptual-cognitive concerns. Ronald is oriented and alert, exhibits good short-term memory, and does not ignore objects on the left that would indicate unilateral neglect. However, his lack of error detection creates safety issues. For example, the quad cane gets in his way during transfers. Since his length of stay is only 3 weeks, a long cognitive test battery is probably not feasible. A thorough evaluation of cognition may be possible during the outpatient phase of his care.

Ronald's concerns gradually surface as the therapist establishes rapport with him. He confides that he is "happy to be getting therapy," because he wants to go home with his wife. He also likes to show young children how to "shoot hoops." Self-care test results suggest a good match between his level of function and his desire to have his wife take care of him at home. However, further information is needed about his "lack of error detection" to decide whether his wife can leave him at home unattended. Because he has impaired arm and trunk control, and balance could not be safely tested, Ronald may not be able to resume playing basketball and doing yardwork. More information about "volunteering at his church" is needed to determine whether Ronald can resume this valued activity. ■

Summary

Selection of appropriate assessments is a complex process that requires the occupational therapist to take into account the needs of the client, the setting for intervention, the environmental and temporal context of the client, and the frame(s) of reference selected to guide treatment and phases of evaluation. Each client presents a unique set of needs, and the therapist must use his or her clinical reasoning skills in the evaluation and intervention process. Ultimately, appropriate assessment selection will provide the therapist with timely reliable and valid information to guide the intervention process.

References

Allen, C.K. (1990). *Allen cognitive level test manual* (with kit included). Colchester, CT: S & S/Worldwide.

American Occupational Therapy Association. (1994). Uniform terminology for occupational therapy (3rd ed.). *American Journal of Occupational Therapy, 48*, 1047–1954.

Ayres, A.J. (1976, March). Clinical observations of neuromuscular integration. Administration of the Southern California Sensory Integration Tests, Certification Course. Conference sponsored by the Center for the Study of Sensory Integrative Dysfunction, held at Valhalla, NY.

Ayres, A.J. (1989). *Sensory integration and praxis tests.* Los Angeles: Western Psychological Services.

Brayman, S.J., & Kirby, T. (1982). Comprehensive occupational therapy evaluation scale. In B. Hemphill (ed.), *The evaluation process in psychiatric occupational therapy* (pp. 211–226). Thorofare, NJ: Slack.

Bruininks, R. (1978). *Bruininks-Oseretsky Test of Motor Proficiency,* Circle Pines, MN: American Guidance Service.

Brunnstrom, S. (1970). *Movement therapy in hemiplegia.* Philadelphia: Harper & Row.

Bundy. A. (1977). *Play and playfulness: What to look for.* In D.L. Parham & L.S. Fazio (Ed.), *Play in occupational therapy for children* (pp. 52–66). St. Louis, MO: Mosby-Year Book.

Cohen, E.S. (1988). The elderly mystique: Constraints on the autonomy of the elderly with disabilities. *Gerontologist, 28*, 29.

Dellon, A. (1988). *Evaluation of sensibility and re-education of sensation of the hand.* Baltimore, MD: Lucas.

Denton, P. (1987). *Psychiatric occupational therapy: A workbook of practical skills.* Boston: Little, Brown & Company.

Dutton, R. (1995). *Clinical reasoning in physical disabilities.* Baltimore: Williams & Wilkins.

Frankenberg, W.K., Dodds, J., Archer, P., Bresnick, B., Maschka, P., Edelman, N., & Shapiro, H. (1991). *The Denver II developmental screening test.* Denver, CO: Denver Developmental Materials.

Furuno, S., O'Reilly, K.A., Hosaka, C.M., Inatsuka, T.T., Allman, T.A., & Zeisloft, B. (1984). *Hawaii Early Learning Profile (HELP).* Palo Alto, CA: Vort Corporation.

Gardner, M.F. (1986). *Test of Visual-Motor Skills (TVMS).* Burlingame, CA: Psychological and Educational Publications.

Hinojosa, J. & Kramer, P. (1997). Integrating children with disabilities into family play. In D.L. Parham & L.S. Fazio (ed.), *Play in occupational therapy for children* (pp. 159–170). St. Louis, MO: Mosby-Year Book.

Itzkovich, M., Elazar, B., & Averbuck, F. (1990). *Lowenstein occupational therapy cognitive assessment.* Pequannock, NJ: Maddak.

Jette, A.M., Davis, A.R., Cleary, P.D., Calkins, D.R., Ruberstein, L.V., Fink, A., Kosecoft, S., Young, R.T., Brook, R.H., & Delbanco, T.L. (1986). The functional status questionnaire:

Reliability and validity when used in primary care. *Journal of General Internal Medicine, 1,* 143–149.

Kielhofner, G. (1985). *A model of human occupation.* Baltimore: Williams & Wilkins.

Kielhofner, G. (1995). *A model of human occupation* (2nd ed.). Baltimore: Williams & Wilkins.

Kielhofner, G., Mallinson, T., de las Heras, C.G. (1995). Methods of data gathering. In G. Kielhofner, *A model of human occupation* (2nd ed.) (pp. 209–214). Baltimore: Williams & Wilkins.

Kohlman-Thompson, L. (1992). *Kohlman evaluation of living skills (KELS)* (3rd ed.). Bethesda, MD: American Occupational Therapy Association.

Leonardelli, C. (1988). *Milwaukee evaluation of daily living skills.* Thorofare, NJ: Slack.

Levine, R. (1988). Community home health. In H.L. Hopkins & H.D. Smith (eds.), *Willard and Spackman's occupational therapy* (7th ed.) (p. 772). Philadelphia: Lippincott.

Matsutsuyu, J.S. (1969). The interest checklist. *American Journal of Occupational Therapy, 23,* 323–328.

Miller, L.J. (1982). *The Miller Assessment for Preschoolers* (MAP). New York, NY: Psychological Corporation.

Miller, L.J. (1993). *Toddler and Infant Motor Evaluation (TIME).* Tucson, AZ: Therapy Skill Builders.

Mutti, M., Sterling, H.M., & Saplding, N.V. (1978). *Quick Neurological Screening Test (QNST).* Novato, CA: Academic Therapy.

Piper, M.C., & Darrah, J. (1994). *Alberta Infant Motor Scales (AIMS).* Philadelphia: W.B. Saunders.

Takata, N. (1974). Play as a prescription. In M. Reilly (Ed.), *Play as exploratory learning.* Beverly Hills, CA: Sage.

Valpar International Corporation. (1986). *Valpar international corporation brochure.* Tuscon, AZ: Valpar International Corporation.

Williams, S.L., & Bloomer, J. (1987). *Bay area functional performance evaluation administration and scoring manual* (2nd ed.). Palo Alto, CA: Consulting Psychologists Press.

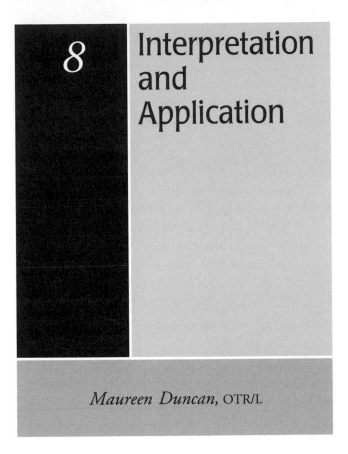

8 Interpretation and Application

Maureen Duncan, OTR/L

Overview

Once occupational therapists have administered various assessments, they become concerned with interpreting the information. This chapter presents the process of interpretation. It describes how occupational therapists interpret information from the assessments that they have administered as well as from observational data gathered throughout the evaluative process. Other factors that influence how that particular data will be interpreted are also outlined. Finally, this chapter discusses the relation between evaluation interpretation and the intervention plan.

Introduction

Many factors influence the evaluation interpretive process, among them the philosophical assumptions of the profession, frame of reference, clinical reasoning skills, knowledge regarding assessment strengths and limitations, the use of additional quantitative and qualitative data, and therapist bias and expectations. In addition, the application of interpretive findings is often guided by organizational goals such as standard protocol and by individual perceptions regarding intervention. The process of interpretation is essential to making sound practice decisions throughout occupational therapy intervention. Evaluation cannot be seen as complete until one has interpreted the evaluative findings that result in clinical decision-making.

The Interpretive Process Continuum

Throughout the data-gathering process, the therapist makes preliminary interpretations based on formal and informal information that may include client history, referral information, observations, interactions with the individual, and results from assessments. As new information is made available, the therapist incorporates this into his or her knowledge base and, through the use of deductive and inductive reasoning, interprets the information to make informed decisions resulting in the development and refinement of intervention plans.

FROM INCEPTION TO DISCHARGE

Interpretation and application of interpretive findings during the evaluative process occur continually from inception to discharge (Medhurst & Ryan, 1996; Parham, 1987; Stewart, 1996). As you will recall from Chapter 1, the Commission on Practice of the American Occupational Therapy Association (AOTA) has defined evaluation to include "planning for and documenting the process, results and recommendations, including the need for intervention and/or potential change in the intervention plan." Therefore, the evaluative process is an integral component in occupational therapy.

The evaluation process consists of obtaining and interpreting data that reflect the individual's current status. This is clearly stated in the AOTA *Standards of Practice* (AOTA, 1994a). Standard IV; Section 6, states that "registered occupational therapists shall analyze and summarize collected evaluation data to indicate the individual's current functional status" (p. 1040). When analyzing data regarding the individual's current status, the therapist should identify both strengths and limitations (Rogers & Holm, 1991).

Interpretation begins early in the evaluation process in the form of a preliminary screening, during which the therapist interprets information gathered and, through the use of clinical reasoning, determines whether a complete occupational therapy evaluation is warranted.

The interpretive process continues well after implementation of the intervention plan. The therapist continually reevaluates the individual's current status by gathering and interpreting information regarding the effectiveness of treatment on occupational performance, thus allowing for changes to be made in the intervention plan when needed.

As professionals, occupational therapists must be able to justify how practice decisions are made. Therefore, interpretations must be based on more than hunches and intuition. Intrepretation is a skill, learned and refined through practice, that is guided by the philosophical assumptions of the profession and by frames of reference.

Guiding Philosophical Assumptions

Intervention planning is grounded in both the domain of concern and the philosophical assumptions of a profession. This is true for occupational therapy as for other professions.

PHILOSOPHICAL BELIEFS OF OCCUPATIONAL THERAPY

The interpretations therapists make during the evaluation process and the practice decisions they arrive at are guided by the assumptions, beliefs, and values of occupational therapy practice. Theoretical beliefs are described by Parham (1987) as "thinking tools for the reflective occupational therapist" (p. 556), because they are used as a guide in clinical decision-making.

Mosey (1981, 1986, 1996) provides us with an excellent example of what guides occupational therapy practice. She contends that a profession is characterized by its philosophical assumptions, ethical code, theoretical foundation, domain of concern, legitimate tools, and the nature of and principles for practice. Some philosophical beliefs of occupational therapy include:

- belief that the individual will meet his or her physical, psychological, and social needs through occupation
- belief that each individual is unique
- belief in autonomy of the individual
- belief that the individual must be viewed holistically
- belief that if given the opportunity, an individual will strive to reach his or her fullest potential.

While occupational therapy practice is based on the philosophical beliefs of the profession, it also follows particular models and frames of reference. This is reflected in the data collection, interpretation, and intervention planning phases of the evaluation process. While this is particularly evident in the intervention phase of evaluation, the effects of models and frames of reference occur throughout the entire process.

THE USE OF FRAMES OF REFERENCE AS A GUIDE IN THE INTERPRETIVE PROCESS

Frame of reference, identified as *delineation* models by Kortman (1994), describe the guiding constructs for assessments and the principles for intervention. Frames of reference delineate a function/dysfunction continuum and behaviors indicative of function and dysfunction, which guide the evaluative process (Kramer & Hinojosa, 1993a).

The frame of reference chosen to aid in guiding the interpretive process is based on the individual client's needs (Kramer & Hinojosa, 1993b), the philosophical beliefs of the therapist (Hinojosa & Kramer, 1993; Mosey, 1981), and the practices of the intervention setting (Mosey, 1981; Muhlenhaupt, 1993; Rogers & Holm, 1991). Frames of reference cannot be used as formulas for action. They are meant to guide therapists only by providing direction for evaluation and intervention (Mosey, 1981, 1996).

The concern of a frame of reference tends to be narrow and to address one area of practice (Mosey, 1981). Therefore, multiple frames of reference may be used to guide the decision-making process in the evaluation of an individual with complex problems (Kramer & Hinojosa, 1993c). Because therapists are often working with complex problems, the task of integrating philosophical beliefs and data may at times be overwhelming. Therapists must have a way of organizing and interpreting information from all aspects of the evaluation in a usable format that results in sound clinical judgments. Frames of reference provide this guideline. The process of interpretation is multidimensional. It involves interpreting data from numerous quantitative and qualitative sources, such as that gathered from standardized and nonstandardized assessments, through skilled observations, from interviews, and from medical and nonmedical records (for example, written narrative).

Factors Influencing Interpretation

Many factors influence the interpretive process. The therapist's use of clinical reasoning, level of expertise, and organizational philosophy all affect how, and in what way, a therapist interprets data.

CLINICAL REASONING

As discussed in Chapter 2, clinical reasoning plays a crucial role in the evaluation process. The process of clinical reasoning is described variously as intensive, dynamic, and multidimensional (Fleming, 1991; Mattingly, 1991a; Munroe, 1996; Robertson, 1996a). "Clinical reasoning is a complex and multidimensional concept encompassing a wide range of cognitive activities which underpin the judgments and decisions made by health professionals in the context of their clinical practice" (Munroe, 1996, p. 196). While therapists often use a dominant form of clinical reasoning, different forms of clinical reasoning may be used during various stages of interpretation (Robertson, 1996a). As we see, the form of clinical reasoning used influences the interpretive process.

Munroe (1996) has identified three primary forms of clinical reasoning commonly found in occupational therapy practice: theory-based clinical reasoning (Parham, 1987); information processing (Rogers & Holm, 1991); and clinical reasoning as a narrative process (Fleming, 1991; Mattingly, 1991a).

According to Munroe (1996), theory-based clinical reasoning and information processing are the dominant views of clinical reasoning in occupational therapy practice. These forms of clinical reasoning fall under the broad category of scientific reasoning, which reflects our tendency as a profession to follow the reductionist medical model, where an emphasis is placed on diagnosis and the following of established treatment protocols. However, while many therapists use problem-solving techniques based on the model of scientific reasoning, many others do not (Fleming, 1991; Schon, 1983). Fleming (1991) identified four types of clinical reasoning used in occupational therapy practice. These include:

1. narrative reasoning, such as described by Mattingly (1991a)
2. procedural reasoning, consisting of "problem identification, goal setting, and treatment planning" (Fleming, 1991, p. 1008)
3. interactive reasoning, "focus[ing] on the phenomenological person as an individual" (Fleming, 1991, p. 1010)
4. conditional reasoning, which takes into consideration the "social and temporal contexts" (Fleming, 1991, p. 1011).

Fleming concluded that "occupational therapists seem to shift smoothly from one mode of thinking to another in order to analyze, interpret, and resolve various types of clinical problems" (p. 1007).

While many forms of clinical reasoning have been identified in the occupational therapy literature, they can generally be broken down into three distinct categories (Schell & Cervero, 1993). Table 8.1 identifies clinical reasoning approaches commonly used in occupational therapy practice.

The interpretation process is strongly influenced by the form of clinical reasoning used throughout evaluation. Therapists who use scientific reasoning are likely to focus on the disease process and the diagnosis of the individual. The assessments they choose and the interpretations they make are based on the hypotheses formed during initial screening. They look for information that will support their hypothesis. Numerous examples of this form of clinical reasoning can be found in occupational therapy practice (Parham, 1987; Rogers, 1983; Rogers & Holm, 1991).

Therapists who use a narrative approach to clinical reasoning spend considerable time gathering information that will allow them to understand how the disease process or diagnosis affects their client. A focus is placed on acquiring knowledge that will accurately represent the unique perspective of the individual. Therapists interpret data that they believe will aid them in

■ *Table 8.1.* Clinical Reasoning Approaches Commonly Used in Occupational Therapy Practice

Category	Definition	Variations and Authors
Scientific reasoning	Systematic cognitive process based on rational thought processes Focus: disease process and/or disability	Diagnostic reasoning (Rogers, 1983) Theory-based reasoning (Rogers & Holm, 1991) Information processing (Parham, 1987)
Narrative reasoning	In order to understand the disease process, one must elicit the individual's story Focus: understanding the disease process from the individual's point of view	Reflection in action (Schon, 1983) Story telling/story making (Mattingly, 1991a, 1991b) Procedural reasoning, interactive reasoning, conditional reasoning (Fleming, 1991)
Pragmatic reasoning	Based on the work of cognitive psychologists, looks at personal and practice constraint such as reimbursement and equipment availability Focus: practical issues surrounding practice	(Barris, 1987; Schell & Cervero, 1993)

gaining information and making decisions that will be in their client's best interest. Procedural, interactive, and conditional reasoning all fall within this category (Fleming, 1991; Mattingly, 1991a; Schon, 1983).

The third broad category of clinical reasoning is known as pragmatic reasoning. This takes into consideration the constraints on occupational therapy imposed by organizational or administrative philosophy, such as time constraints, space and equipment availability, and reimbursement. Pragmatic reasoning influences the interpretive process in several ways. When therapists are limited in the amount of time they have to complete an evaluation, they focus on interpreting data that will yield the greatest amount of information in the shortest amount of time. This may mean interpreting sections of standardized tests that address their client's specific area of limitation, rather than scoring and interpreting the entire assessment. Therapists may also focus on interpreting data that are needed for documentation and subsequent reimbursement of services. Reimbursement often hinges on objective data that justify the need for intervention. Therefore, interpreting subjective data may not be seen as valuable (Barris, 1987; Schell & Cervero, 1993).

These three broad categories of clinical reasoning are not mutually exclusive. Occupational therapists often use more than one form of reasoning. For example, Fleming (1991) uses a blending of narrative and pragmatic reasoning.

Clinical reasoning can be identified by method (scientific reasoning, narrative reasoning, or pragmatic reasoning) and by style (deductive or inductive reasoning).

DEDUCTIVE AND INDUCTIVE REASONING

The clinical reasoning used in the interpretation and application phase of evaluation can be viewed as both deductive and inductive in nature (Rogers, 1983). Deductive reasoning is a logical process that begins with the generation of a hypothesis based on very specific principles. This form of reasoning parallels that of scientific reasoning and is most often used by medical professionals.

Inductive reasoning is a logical process in which hypotheses or generalizations are formed based on observations and facts. Inductive reasoning used during the interpretive process helps to guide the focus of intervention. It begins with the therapist asking "What if?" questions. As each piece of data is interpreted, it is integrated with previous data to guide decision-making. Therapists do not enter into the interpretive process with preconceived beliefs as to what they are likely to find, as one would when using deductive reasoning. With inductive reasoning, conclusions are only made after the data are interpreted and integrated. This form of reasoning closely parallels that of narrative reasoning (Fleming, 1991; Mattingly, 1991a, 1991b; Schon, 1983).

While therapists often use more than one type of clinical reasoning (for example, narrative and pragmatic), their style of reasoning (deductive versus inductive) is likely to remain constant throughout the interpretive process. As we will see, reasoning style is strongly influenced by level of clinical expertise.

NOVICE/EXPERT

When developing an intervention plan, experience provides the therapist with a knowledge base that can be used to make judgments about the relative importance of the information gathered (Robertson, 1996a). Embrey (1993) found that experienced therapists are more client-oriented, whereas inexperienced therapists are more activity–oriented. Inexperienced therapists are more likely to let knowledge obtained from their academic education guide their decision-making. Entry-level therapists are thus more likely to rely on the use of analytical or scientific decision-making and more likely to persist in the implementation of intervention based on established protocols. Dutton (1995) describes the novice as one who typically rigidly applies rules and principles learned in school. However, as therapists gain skills and experience, their "actions" become smooth, flexible, and spontaneous, and . . . thinking becomes automatic (Rogers, 1983, p. 614).

While novices are able to generate the same number of hypotheses, experts can more accurately interpret and form linkages among data, resulting in an increased understanding of the impact a disability or impairment has on the life of their client (Neistadt, 1996; Robertson, 1996a). The pairing of inexperienced with experienced therapists has been advocated to aid in developing clinical decision-making skills that are based on client-directed needs, as opposed to organizational or practice setting-based goals and objectives (Jensen, Shepard, & Hack, 1990).

ORGANIZATIONAL PHILOSOPHY/ADMINISTRATIVE REGULATIONS

As previously mentioned, therapists are often limited as to what they can or cannot do by the restrictions imposed on them by the practice setting. Organizational philosophy will often stipulate the frame of reference a therapist must use in treatment (Barris, 1987; Rogers & Holm, 1991). This is commonly seen in large facilities which often follow a particular frame of reference, thereby restricting the therapist's scope of practice. An emphasis is often placed on addressing specific performance components with a primary predefined focus. Little emphasis is placed on occupational performance outside of that focus and there is only limited consideration of performance context. Instead, therapists administer and interpret assessments dictated by the practice setting and develop generic intervention plans that are slightly adapted to meet the needs of their clients.

Interventions often fail if based solely on technical skills and procedures, which are narrow in scope, because they fail to look at the broader context. "The outcomes of therapeutic efforts . . . are jeopardized when standard technical solutions are routinely selected without reflection on the scope of the problems faced by the [individual]" (Parham, 1987, p. 556). The application of interpretive findings must address all areas of concern. Applying technical skills alone, without thought to the total individual, is the equivalent of treating only one small piece of the problem (Parham, 1987). While clients may come to us with a diagnosis we have seen and treated on numerous occasions, no two individuals are exactly alike. Each has a unique set of circumstances surrounding his or her disability, which cannot be addressed by the application of a standard protocol. In order to address unique needs of our clients, the interpretation of clinical data must be handled competently and professionally.

Interpretation of Assessment Results/Scores

Some of the following information reviews that presented in previous chapters, because knowledge of how test results influence intrepretation is essential. In many cases, the therapist must interpret data and make clinical decisions based on inconclusive or missing data (Rogers & Holm, 1991). Care must be taken when evaluating noncommunicating adults, dealing with partial records and/ or conflicting data, and deviating from standardized testing.

COMPARING RESULTS TO A NORMATIVE BASE

Scores from norm-referenced tests compare the performance of an individual to that of others: a normative sample. This is expressed in the form of normative data. Norms represent what scores are average or should be anticipated when testing a normal population. During the interpretive process, scores obtained on a standardized instrument are compared to those scores of the normative sample (Asher, 1996; Kaplan, 1996; Paul, 1995).

CRITERION-REFERENCED TESTS

Scores from criterion-referenced tests compare an individual's performance to an external standard of performance (Asher, 1996). This is expressed in the form of a performance criterion. Criterion-referenced test scores reflect the individual's current ability level. The scores on criterion-referenced tests are representative of what the individual can and cannot do. Judgments are then made regarding whether the performance of the individual is adequate or inadequate (e.g., can the individual get in and out of the bathtub safely?).

VALIDITY

As you recall, validity refers to how well a test measures what it is intended to measure. According to Asher (1996), standardized instruments (whether standardized tests, standardized interviews, or standardized observations) consist of standardized procedures, scoring, or apparatus, which must be used precisely throughout the assessment procedure to ensure reliability and validity. "The reliability and validity of the therapist's conclusions are only as good as the reliability and validity of the instrument" (Asher, 1996, p. xxvi). Care must be taken to interpret these results with caution.

Therapist often overlook the fact that administration of standardized tests must follow strict procedures (Kaplan, 1996). When therapists deviate from standard procedural protocol, then normative information cannot be used. This is not to say that the results are useless; the information gained will aid in clinical decision-making. While the test results no longer reflect performance that can be compared to a normative sample, they do reflect performance on specific tasks. However, these results must be interpreted cautiously and should never be used independently of data gathered from other sources which confirm or disconfirm the findings. Furthermore, when standardized procedures are deviated from, scores from results must be reported in a descriptive form that clearly indicates that results are not based on normative data. The AOTA *Standards of Practice* (1994a) states that "if standardized tests are not available or appropriate, the results shall be expressed in descriptive reports, and standardized scales shall not be used" (p. 1040).

The interpretation of standardized test scores must be conducted effectively and ethically. Therapists must have an understanding of statistical and measurement concepts and be experienced in test administration protocol (Kaplan, 1996). In order for therapists to interpret assessment results accurately, resulting in sound clinical judgments, they must understand the relationship between the test scores and conclusion derived from them (Asher, 1996).

TEST BIAS

Occupational therapists should use assessment instruments that are individualized and sensitive to the varying needs and situations of their clients (Pollock, 1993). When interpreting test results, the therapist must take into consideration the norms, values, and beliefs of the individual whose score is being interpreted.

Cultural bias of tests is critical to consider in the interpretation process. In reference to Van de Vijver & Poortinga's work (1991), Paul (1995) concludes that the bias in assessments is not embedded in the instrument, but in the interpretation of the scores as absolute measures. Therapists must be knowledgeable about their client's culture in order to decrease the possibility of misinterpretation (Paul, 1995). Therapists can minimize bias when interpreting assessment results, by increasing their knowledge of cultural differences and by involving the individual in the evaluation process.

Interpretation of both quantitative and qualitative data must take into consideration variations in locus of control, self-determination, and orientation to space and time due to cultural differences. Paul (1995) states that "occupational therapists face new challenges in assessment and treatment planning with clients who do not share with a therapist a common language, differ in health-related beliefs and values, and have different understanding of the nature of work, leisure, and self-care" (p. 156).

When interpreting assessments, the culture of the client plays an important role in the interpretation of the data (Paul, 1995). Many of occupational therapy's assessment tools are developed and based on white middle-class values. The profession of occupational therapy has incorporated these values into its knowledge base, which is reflected in both theory and practice. Using assessments standardized on white middle–class populations with other populations can result in inaccurate interpretation of the scores (Paul, 1995). For example, white middle-class Americans value independence. Occupational therapists place a large amount of emphasis on this and often use the measure of degree of functional independence as an indicator of quality of life and intervention success. For some cultures, such as Asian Americans, and for some individuals with chronic disabilities, such as spinal cord injury (Whalley Hammell, 1995), little emphasis is placed on independence. For these reasons it is important to understand the meaning that "disability" has from the individual's perspective (Mattingly, 1991b).

This is not to say that assessments that use white middle-class Americans as the norm should not be adapted for use to allow for cultural differences.

But cultural differences must be taken into consideration when interpreting test results.

LINKING RESULTS TO OCCUPATIONAL PERFORMANCE

The goal of interpreting data is to "indicate the individual's current functional status" (AOTA, 1994a, p. 1040) so that appropriate interventions can be planned and implemented. The results of interpretations should present a clear picture of the individual's current level of functioning, which includes a description of the individual's strengths and weaknesses. Furthermore, interpretation should reflect the interrelatedness of occupational therapy's domain of concern. This includes a description of performance areas, performance components, and performance context as these apply to the individual's ability to engage in occupations. Test results should never be considered in isolation. They must be confirmed or disconfirmed by other sources of data to reflect a holistic view of the individual. When interpreting test results, the therapist must be aware that results only reflect what the individual is capable of doing on a given day and time under testing circumstances. Test scores cannot by themselves tell us why the individual performs as he or she does (Paul, 1995). Interpretive findings should reflect the domain of concern of occupational therapy practice. Therapists should place their primary area of emphasis on how the findings relate to the individual's ability to engage in functional, everyday activities which they identify as meaningful.

Limitations: Cautions and Precautions

Missing data, incomplete records, test bias, and restrictions imposed by the practice setting on the amount and content of data collected, complicate the interpretive process. Rogers (1983) sums this up in the following way: "Clinical problems are not neat. They are messy and complex. Everything that could be known about the patient is not known and much of the data collected is flawed and imperfect" (p. 614).

INTEGRATION OF QUANTITATIVE AND QUALITATIVE DATA: COMBINING NUMEROUS DATA SOURCES

In keeping with the philosophy of occupational therapy, interpretation must reflect a holistic perspective of the individual and therefore must be completed in a comprehensive manner. Interpretation of evaluation should yield information pertaining to every facet of the individual, outlining both strengths and weakness (Rogers & Holm, 1991). Therefore, interpretation must be based on qualitative, as well as quantitative information. These results will be both objective and subjective in nature (Asher, 1996; Nelson, 1997). Information from objective and subjective sources is used to corroborate findings and formulate conclusions (Asher, 1996).

Clinical decision-making involves combining and interpreting both qualitative and quantitative data from a variety of sources. When determining what data to include in the evaluation, one must ask the question: Do the data fit within the domain of concern of occupational therapy practice? Beginning therapists often ask how much data to gather and interpret. While there are no set guidelines, therapists must gather enough information to present an accurate picture of the client's functional ability. Therapists should keep in mind that the more information they collect, the more they will have to interpret, thus increasing the likelihood of misinterpretation (Rogers & Holm, 1991). When interpreting large amounts of data, therapists are often tempted to sort the data into distinct categories (for example, according to performance components). Robertson (1996b) warns against sorting data from quantitative and qualitative sources into specific categories or areas of concern. Interpretation from data must be integrated to reflect the complex nature of human variability.

The integration of data from a variety of sources can be quite challenging. Therapists must be careful not to make leaps of logic during the interpretive phase. This is likely to occur if data are only gathered from limited sources of information. The use of more than one assessment instrument will aid in eliminating bias. Likewise, therapists should not overinterpret data or interpret data that focus solely on evaluating individual dysfunction, as opposed to function (Rogers, 1983).

THERAPIST BIAS AND EXPECTATION

In Chapter 2, Kramer and Hinojosa warn us to keep information from client histories and charts separate from our own data-gathering and conclusions. Preconceived beliefs will affect both assessment choice and data interpretation. However, preencounter information may be useful under certain circumstances (Rogers & Holm, 1991). During a screening, therapists often base decisions on the limited information that is available at the time. This may include a review of the individual's past medical records and the written diagnosis and prognosis that came with the referral. However, once it has been determined that a full evaluation is warranted, therapists should be aware that this preencounter information may alter their expectations and beliefs regarding appropriate interpretations and intervention strategies. Charts often contain inaccurate or incomplete information. Generating a hypothesis based on preencounter information will restrict or narrow the focus of data collection, which ultimately affects the clinical decisions based on interpretive findings.

To make clinical judgments based on the results of interpretations from limited data is not only unprofessional, but unethical. Principle 3, Section D of the *Occupational Therapy Code of Ethics* (AOTA, 1994b), specifically states that occupational therapists "shall perform their duties on the basis of accurate and current information" (p. 1037). This is discussed further in Chapter 11.

Relationship Between Interpretation and Intervention

Therapists must reflect not only on individual clinical problems, but on the potential outcome of intervention strategies (Schon, 1983). In addition, intervention decisions must be based on clinical reasoning to ensure that individuals receive the highest quality service and that negative consequences are avoided (Rogers, 1983).

Throughout the evaluation process, documentation of findings from assessments, both qualitative and quantitative, as well as documentation of clinical reasoning, must be strictly adhered to. A major element involved in interpretation relates to the therapist's ability to sort through both qualitative and quantitative information, which includes assessment results, context, interpretations and perceptions of the individual, and past knowledge, and identify the focus on intervention plan. Parham (1987) refers to this process as *problem-setting*. She believes that once the problem has been set, the intervention plan can be developed.

CLINICAL DECISION-MAKING

Occupational therapists use "clinical reasoning skills to collect and transform data about [individuals] into decisions that have critical implications for the quality of life of their patients" (Rogers, 1983, p. 601). It is easy to get caught up in the medical clinical decision-making model. Thus, occupational therapists often rely on this form of decision-making to guide treatment or intervention (Mattingly, 1991b). When specific protocols are followed based on a diagnosis, this contributes to the fragmentation of not only the profession of occupational therapy, but also to the intervention strategies employed. Furthermore, it limits the therapist to the needs specified by a diagnosis, rather than giving appropriate attention to the needs of the individual.

Case Example

JESSIE

Beth, an occupational therapist working in a large acute care setting, has just received a referral from Dr. Jones to evaluate and treat a patient (Jessie) for decreased range of motion of the upper extremities. After reviewing Jessie's chart, Beth discovers that Jessie, who is 22, is a patient in the hospital's bone marrow transplant unit and has just undergone 14 days of intensive chemotherapy treatment. During this time, Jessie remained in her bed, gradually growing weaker. Beth visits Jessie that afternoon. When she enters the room she sees a woman lying propped in bed with a kerchief wrapped tightly around her head. A few strands of hair are hanging from one side. Beth introduces herself and, using a goniometer, proceeds to take range of motion measurements. Her preliminary findings suggest that Jessie's range of motion has decreased, but in all likelihood it is still within functional limits. She needs to wait until she returns to the clinic and compares her measurements with the standardized norms before she decides on a treatment plan.

When Beth finishes taking her measurements, Jessie asks Beth if she would bring her a mirror or help her walk to the bathroom so she could see herself. She tells Beth that she has always taken pride in her appearance and is not yet used to the idea of not wearing makeup or having her hair brushed. Jessie tells Beth that she had asked the nurses to help her, but they had insisted she remain in bed until she felt stronger. Beth assures Jessie that she will speak with the nurses and her doctor to determine when Jessie can be up and walking, and in the meantime, she promises to find a hand-held mirror, so that Jessie can apply makeup in bed if she so desires. She tells Jessie that she will be back the following day to begin range of motion exercises and then leaves the room. On her way out, Beth notices a bedside table tray located near the foot of the bed and opens the top to reveal a mirror. She pushes the tray up to the head of the bed and tells Jessie, who is drifting off to sleep, that there is a mirror inside. She quietly says goodbye and leaves. Later that afternoon, Beth sits down to document her evaluative findings.

Beth records her goniometer readings for each of the joints measured and then compares these with those of the normative data. Her findings indicate that Jessie's range of motion is significantly decreased. Based on her assessment results, she establishes the following treatment plan: Range of motion exercises will begin the following morning and be carried out daily. Beth will also teach these exercises to Jessie's parents, who visit daily. This will ensure that Jessie receives range of motion exercise at least two times daily. She will also teach self range of motion exercises to Jessie as soon as her strength and endurance increase enough to allow this. Beth writes the following long- and short-term goals:

Long-Term Goal: Patient will receive UE range of motion 2× daily to increase functional range of motion.

Short-Term Goal: Patient will increase range of motion, by participating in range of motion exercises, by 5 degrees in all planes of motion of upper extremity by January 13.

When she finishes, Beth faxes a copy of her findings, along with her treatment plan, to Dr. Jones. ∎

As you can see, Beth followed standard departmental procedures. After being given a referral for evaluation and treatment of range of motion, and performing an initial chart review, Beth evaluated Jessie's range of motion using a standardized instrument (goniometer). Based on assessment results interpreted by comparing Jessie's measurements to standardized norms, Beth designed an intervention plan to address Jessie's decreased range of motion. This was congruent with the philosophical beliefs of the clinical setting and the frames of reference (biomechanical and neurorehabilitative) used in her department, both of which focus on addressing the performance component deficits.

As an occupational therapist, Beth failed to take into account other factors that should have been considered after reviewing Jessie's chart, observing Jessie's weakened appearance, and speaking directly with Jessie regarding her desire to view her image in a mirror. Data from each of these sources should have been integrated into the evaluation and interpretation process, so that performance areas, other performance components, and performance context were at a minimum considered in the treatment plan. Instead, a standard protocol was followed to evaluate a diagnostic specific problem area. Clinical decision-making in this case was strongly influenced by the amount and type of information that Beth allowed herself to consider during the interpretive process.

During the process of clinical decision-making, the therapist must determine what additional information is needed to make sound clinical judgments. Principle 3, Section G of the *Code of Ethics* (1994b) requires occupational therapists to "consult with other service providers when additional knowledge and expertise is required" (p. 1038). When information is incomplete or when additional information is needed, the therapist must seek out information from individuals who are knowledgeable in the area being addressed.

In the above case example, Beth should have consulted with physical therapy (to determine whether they were addressing the patient's decreased strength and endurance, and desire to walk), with the physician and psychologist (to learn more about Jessie's responses to chemotherapy), and most importantly, with Jessie's family (to determine what meaning the disease process held for them and what their personal goals were for intervention).

SELF-MONITORING

Clinical decision-making rests in part on the therapist's ability to reflect on past experiences and apply this information to the current situation. This "reflection in action" occurs throughout the evaluation (Schon, 1983). Therapists interpret findings based on a combination of available data, tacit knowledge, and past experience. Past experience aids the therapist in determining what information is important and what is irrelevant (Robertson, 1996a).

Munroe (1996) found that reflection in action was commonly used by therapists in home health care and that "reasoning was relativistic and prognostic in response to contextual influences" (p. 198). This was thought to be due in part to the autonomous role of occupational therapists in community-based practice arenas, such as home health. Therapists who practice autonomously are often put in the position of making quick clinical decisions. These decisions must be based on the therapist's current knowledge and experience and on knowledge of the available resources and influences of the environment (Robertson, 1996b). Under these conditions, therapists often rely on intuitive and reflective thinking in action to guide clinical decision-making (Munroe, 1996).

"The selection of goals and methods for intervention always brings ethical concerns and value judgments into the picture" (Parham, 1987, p. 558). According to Rogers (1983), the most important question to be answered during clinical decision-making is, "What, among the many things that could be done for this patient, ought to be done?" (p. 602). Organizational philosophy and frames of reference are often used to aid in answering this question by providing direction for the selection of goals and the development of intervention plans.

THERAPIST'S RATIONALE—BASED ON INTERPRETATION

Clinical decision-making based on evaluation is, by its very nature, setting-specific. The therapist is expected to relay interpretive findings clearly and concisely following clinical setting guidelines. Information regarding clinical decision-making must be understood by other team members, reviewers, and internal and external audits. Therapists must be able to justify the need for occupational therapy intervention and must convince others that what they do is necessary for increasing client function. "Professional thinking involves being able to clearly and critically analyze the reasons for the decisions and actions we take" (Parham, 1987, p. 155).

Information must also be made available to the individual and his or her designated representatives including family, caregivers, and other professionals (Chapter 11 will provide complete details on the disclosure of confidential information). The communication of interpretive information should be audience-appropriate and presented in an understandable format. Clinical findings should be documented in such a way (following established documentation format) as to ensure that all team members can easily read and understand the content. When transmitting information to individuals, families, and caregivers, language must be free from clinical jargon. The use of acronyms, such as UE and ROM, should be clearly defined. In addition, therapists must document their rationale when making changes to the intervention plan.

Changes in intervention strategies can and should be made whenever new information emerges. For example, new information shared during team meetings can be integrated into the therapist's current knowledge base regarding the individual. Intervention strategies are ultimately based on the therapist's interpretation through clinical decision-making. However, the individual's perspective of the specific situation and how it will affect him or her personally must be given appropriate attention. Individual concerns are not treated as separate pieces of data. They are integrated and incorporated into the interpretation and application phase of intervention (Robertson, 1991b).

INDIVIDUALS AS ACTIVE PARTICIPANTS IN APPLICATION/INTERVENTION PLANNING

Application of interpretive findings, regardless of how good the therapist's intentions, will fail to meet the client's needs if his or her own concerns are not taken into consideration. Decision-making must reflect not only interpretive findings, but the individual's concerns and expectations for outcome. Decision-making is therefore considered to be uniquely individualized (Rogers, 1983). Each individual brings a unique perspective to the situation and should be given the opportunity to express his or her concerns and expectations regarding intervention. Furthermore, throughout the interpretive process, individuals should be allowed to provide input that they feel is beneficial to the final intervention plan (Mattingly, 1991b; Pollock, 1993; Rogers, 1983). This information should be incorporated into the therapist's clinical decision-making at all levels of evaluation. Finally, the therapist should be aware of his or her own biases and be sure that they do not interfere with the decision-making and intervention-planning process.

Summary

Evaluation is concerned with the domain of concern of occupational therapy, as delineated by AOTA's Uniform Terminology (1994c). This consists of performance areas, performance components, and performance context. Interpretation of data from all three domains must be consistent with the philosophical beliefs and assumptions of occupational therapy. While frames of reference guide evaluation, including interpretation and application of findings, they do not stand alone in the clinical decision-making process. The needs of the client and setting should be taken into account and included in the process.

Interpretation of evaluative findings from standardized and nonstandardized assessments must be performed continuously. When interpreting test results, occupational therapists must have a full understanding of normative data, in order to make meaningful decisions and comparisons. Clinical judgments should not be made based on test scores alone. Therefore, therapists must ensure that data they interpret come from a variety of quantitative and qualitative sources. An emphasis should be placed on allowing the individual to take an active role during the interpretive and intervention-planning process.

Lastly, care must be taken to minimize sociocultural and therapist bias. This can be accomplished by the therapist becoming knowledgeable of various cultures and by being aware that standardized and nonstandardized tests are often culturally biased, as well as by having a strong awareness of one's own assumptions and biases.

References

American Occupational Therapy Association. (1993). Occupational therapy roles. *American Journal of Occupational Therapy, 47,* 1087–1105.

American Occupational Therapy Association. (1994a). Standards of practice for occupational therapy. *American Journal of Occupational Therapy, 48,* 1039–1043.

American Occupational Therapy Association. (1994b). Occupational therapy code of ethics. *American Journal of Occupational Therapy, 48,* 1037–1038.

American Occupational Therapy Association. (1994c). Uniform terminology for occupational therapy (3rd ed.). *American Journal of Occupational Therapy, 48,* 1047–1054.

Asher, I.E. (1996). *Occupational therapy assessment tools: An annotated index,* (3rd ed.). Bethesda, MD: American Occupational Therapy Association.

Barris, R. (1987). Clinical reasoning in psychosocial occupational therapy. *Occupational Therapy Journal of Research, 7,* 147–162.

Dutton, R. (1995). *Clinical reasoning in physical disabilities.* Baltimore: Williams & Wilkins.

Embrey, D.G. (1993). Clinical decision making in novice and experienced pediatric physical therapists [Abstract]. *Pediatric Physical Therapy, 5, (4),* 193.

Embrey, D.G., Guthrie, M.R., White, O.R., & Dietz, J. (1996). Clinical decision making by experienced and inexperienced pediatric occupational therapists for children with diplegic cerebral palsy. *Physical Therapy, 76, (1),* 20–33.

Fleming, M.H. (1991). The therapist with the three-track mind. *American Journal of Occupational Therapy, 45,* 1007–1014.

Jensen, G.M., Shepard, K.F., & Hack, L.M. (1990). The novice versus the experienced clinician: Insights into the work of physical therapists. *Physical Therapy, 70,* 314–323.

Hinojosa, J., & Kramer, P. (1993). From frames of reference to actual intervention. In P. Kramer & J. Hinojosa (Eds.), *Frames of reference for occupational therapy* (pp. 439–545). Baltimore: Williams & Wilkins.

Kaplan, S. (1996). Clinical evaluation of standardized tests. *Occupational Therapy in Health Care, 10, (3),* 3–14.

Kortman, B. (1994). The eye of the beholder: Models in occupational therapy. *Australian Occupational Therapy Journal, 41,* 115–122.

Kramer, P., & Hinojosa, J. (1993a). Structure of the frame of reference. In P. Kramer & J. Hinojosa (Eds.), *Frames of reference for occupational therapy* (pp. 37–48). Baltimore: Williams & Wilkins.

Kramer, P., & Hinojosa, J. (1993b). Influence of the human context on the application of frames of reference. In P. Kramer & J. Hinojosa (Eds.), *Frames of reference for occupational therapy* (pp. 475–482). Baltimore: Williams & Wilkins.

Kramer, P., & Hinojosa, J. (1993c). Alternative applications of frames of reference. In P. Kramer & J. Hinojosa (Eds.), *Frames of reference for occupational therapy* (pp. 447–454). Baltimore: Williams & Wilkins.

Lawson, M.J. (1984). Being executive about metacognition. In J.R. Kirby (Ed.), *Cognitive strategies and education performance*. New York: Academic Press.

Mattingly, C. (1991a). The narrative nature of clinical reasoning. *American Journal of Occupational Therapy, 45,* 998–1005.

Mattingly, C. (1991b). What is clinical reasoning? *American Journal of Occupational Therapy, 45,* 979–986.

Medhurst, A., & Ryan, S. (1996). Clinical reasoning in local authority paediatric occupational therapy: Planning a major adaptation for the child with a degenerative condition, Part 2. *British Journal of Occupational Therapy, 59, (6),* 269–272.

Mosey, A.C. (1981). *Occupational therapy: Configuration of a profession.* New York: Raven Press.

Mosey, A.C. (1986). *Psychosocial components of occupational therapy.* New York: Raven Press.

Mosey, A.C. (1996). *Applied scientific inquiry in the health professions: An epistemological orientation* (2nd ed.). Bethesda, MD: American Occupational Therapy Association.

Muhlenhaupt, M. (1993). Influence of settings on the application of frames of reference. In P. Kramer & J. Hinojosa (Eds.), *Frames of reference for occupational therapy* (pp. 455–473). Baltimore: Williams & Wilkins.

Munroe, H. (1996). Clinical reasoning in community occupational therapy. *British Journal of Occupational Therapy, 59, (5),* 196–202.

Neistadt, M.E. (1996). Clinical reasoning in community occupational therapy. *British Journal of Occupational Therapy, 59, (5),* 196–202.

Nelson, D.L. (1997). Why the profession of occupational therapy will flourish in the 21st century: The Eleanor Clarke Slagle Lecture. *American Journal of Occupational Therapy, 51,* 11–24.

Parham, D. (1987). Toward professionalism: The reflective therapist. Nationally Speaking. *American Journal of Occupational Therapy, 41,* 555–561.

Paul, S. (1995). Culture and its influence on occupational therapy evaluation. *Canadian Journal of Occupational Therapy, 62, (3),* 154–161.

Pollock, N. (1993). Client-centered assessment. *American Journal of Occupational Therapy, 47,* 298–301.

Roberts, A.E. (1996). Clinical reasoning in occupational therapy: Idiosyncrasies in content and process. *British Journal of Occupational Therapy, 59, (8),* 372–376.

Robertson, L.J. (1996a). Clinical reasoning, Part 1: The nature of problem solving, a literature review. *British Journal of Occupational Therapy, 59, (8),* 372–376.

Robertson, L.J. (1996b). Clinical reasoning, Part 2: Novice/expert differences. *British Journal of Occupational Therapy, 59, (5),* 212–216.

Rogers, J.C. (1983). Clinical reasoning: The ethics, science, and art. The Eleanor Clarke Slagle Lectureship, 1983. *American Journal of Occupational Therapy, 32,* 601–616.

Rogers, J.C., & Holm, M.B. (1991). Occupational therapy diagnostic reasoning: A component of clinical reasoning. *American Journal of Occupational Therapy, 45,* 1045–1053.

Schell, B.A., & Cervero, R.M. (1993). Clinical reasoning in occupational therapy: An integrative review. *American Journal of Occupational Therapy, 47,* 605–610.

Schon, D.A. (1983). *The reflective practitioner: How professionals think in action.* New York: Basic Books.

Stewart, K.B. (1996). Occupational therapy assessments in pediatrics: Purposes, process, and methods of evaluation. In J. Case-Smith, A.S. Allen, & P.N. Pratt (Eds.), *Occupational therapy for children* (3rd ed.) (pp. 165–199). St. Louis, MO: Mosby.

Van de Vijver, F.J., & Poortinga, Y.H. (1991). Testing across cultures. In R.K. Hambleton & J.N. Zaal (Eds.), *Advances in educational and psychological testing: Theory and application.* Boston: Kluwer Academic.

Whalley Hammell, K. (1995). Spinal cord injury; quality of life; occupational therapy: Is there a connection? *British Journal of Occupational Therapy, 58, (4),* 151–157.

9 Documentation

Cynthia Hughes Harris, PHD, OTR, FAOTA

Overview

In this chapter, the elements of documentation will be explored. The formal purposes of the documenting process will be discussed, as will actual procedures of documentation. As various service delivery systems develop and evolve into greater levels of complexity, occupational therapy practitioners must be attuned to the importance and implications of documentation. Towards that end, types of documentation, the content of documentation notes, and advantages and disadvantages of documentation formats will also be addressed. It would be remiss to omit a discussion of methods of effective documentation, including the importance of good writing. Frequently, information resulting from an interaction between practitioner and client is lost because of poor documentation skills. This chapter will provide a basis for increasing one's understanding of what documentation is, how it is used, and how to do it, so that all intervention interactions are accurately recorded for maximum utilization by others.

Introduction

It has been established in previous chapters that evaluation and assessment are critical aspects of the occupational therapy intervention process. The importance of the documentation process cannot be minimized. Without documentation, the other components of the intervention cycle, including evaluation, are rendered meaningless. It is documentation that confirms that an occupational therapy intervention actually occurred; it is documentation that solidifies the intervention by making the therapeutic process reportable and therefore real; and it is documentation that clearly states or presents the professional judgment and decision-making of the occupational therapy practitioner.

Relative to the multitude of professional responsibilities, documentation must be particularly emphasized, because it is through documentation that the members of the service provision community gain access to the principles, purposes, and propositions of occupational therapy. In addition to documentation being a direct report of the results of practitioner-client interactions, documentation also serves to communicate what we do, why we do it, and who benefits from our services. Simply stated, "documentation is one of the most important functions performed by occupational therapists" (Perinchief, 1993, p. 387).

Documentation can be viewed as evidence or verification of a professional interaction between the practitioner and the client. In some ways, the process of documenting is an information-handling technique. It allows the practitioner to sort, organize, and draw conclusions about the client's status, level of functioning, and therapeutic needs. Documentation facilitates the ability of the occupational therapy practitioner to break down not only the steps but also the concepts of therapy, into more easily understood components. The more the process of therapy is understood, the more meaningful it is, not only to the client, but also to other team members. Documentation reveals what is known and frequently what still has to be learned or accomplished. Therefore, good documentation, meaning a well-written, organized, logically presented record, can lead to increased understanding of the professional perspective of the occupational therapy practitioner, as well as increased respect from others about the role of occupational therapy in the intervention process.

Purposes

There has always been an expectation that occupational therapy practitioners *should*, in some form or fashion, record the process and results of their interventions. The expectation in today's world is that practitioners *must* record their findings. The expectations of documentation are so high that professional survival is dependent on consistent, accurate, and relevant documentation. The legal, ethical, and financial implications of documentation provide the basis for understanding the specific purposes of the process. Of the multiple reasons why occupational therapy practitioners and all other professionals document the results of their professional interventions, the primary ones are as follows:

1. *To serve as the primary path of communication between professionals.* It is the communication component of documentation that gives the practitioner what Denton describes as "interdisciplinary credibility" (Denton, 1987, p. 166). All other team members have access to the practitioner's notes. The physician, physical therapist, social worker, nurse, pharmacist, teacher, psychologist, administrator, third-party payer, and others use the content of the occupational therapy note to gain information about the client's involvement in therapy. As a result, any one of them might change, modify, or confirm the course of his or her own interaction with the client, based on the content of the practitioner's note. The documentation note facilitates linkages among members of the team and their respective goals. Additionally, those same individuals increase their understanding of the role and contribution of occupational therapy. A side effect of good note writing is the potential for an increase in the appropriate use of occupational therapy services with other clients.

2. *To serve as a record of client transactions by caregivers.* Notes are one of the major sources, and in most cases the only source, about what transpired between the practitioner and the client. "The documentation record provides a chronological and ordered record of the complete course of therapeutic intervention" (AOTA, 1994, p. 1). It is no wonder that notes written by professionals are viewed as legal documents. Documented notes can reveal the performance status of the client, the occupational therapy practitioner's plan to affect that status, what the practitioner actually does with the client, and how the client responds to the therapeutic intervention. Through documented records, both the rights of the client and the rights of the practitioner are protected.

3. *To serve as a justification of the process of intervention.* Today, more than ever before in the history of health care, decisions regarding medical care and treatment are being influenced by third-party payers such as Medicare reviewers and representatives from insurance companies, as they engage in determinations regarding reimbursement for services. It is the practitioner's note that justifies the need for occupational therapy services and provides the basis for many reimbursement decisions. The note functions as a gauge that measures appropriateness, effectiveness, and necessity of intervention services. Critical decisions can be

influenced by the quality and completeness of the note. Similarly, in schools and community programs, documentation notes can provide an explanation of the educational relevance of occupational therapy services and a clear understanding of why these services are important and necessary.

4. *Documentation serves to facilitate effective intervention.* A good documentation record reflects the thinking, reasoning, and clinical decision-making of the occupational therapy practitioner. A good note also requires organization and logical thinking on the part of the practitioner. As the practitioner engages in the intervention process, a link is established between the interaction with the client and the documentation of the interaction. As a result, the logic of the documentation influences the clinical reasoning of the interactions. To think in an organized manner for documentation purposes affects the planning and problem-solving of the intervention process. Therefore, a logical documentation approach can structure thinking for client-related problem solving.

5. *Documentation serves as a basis for research.* Again, now more than ever before, occupational therapists are identifying research opportunities within the realm of their daily practice. As documentation has increased in importance and the need for timely, accurate, and relevant notes has become the minimum standard for practice, the research potential of documented notes has increased significantly. The documented note is now the basis for efficacy and outcome studies. Data from the notes can be collected, resulting in both hypotheses and conclusions generated about the types of clients and the types of interventions that were employed. As the need for meaningful documentation practices continues to increase in importance and as documentation standards increase, it is expected that more therapists will view documentation records as prospective research data and will write documentation notes with research as a goal.

For the most part, occupational therapy practitioners document in order to achieve one of the above purposes. Those who deviate from these purposes into arenas that address their personal needs and interests, severely compromise the impact of the documentation. If the designated purposes of documentation are ignored, then the impact of documentation is lost.

Types of Documentation

Documentation can refer to either the means of recording the content, as in documentation delivery, or to the categories of documentation relative to the type of content being documented. When addressing documentation delivery, two approaches are used: paper-based systems and computer-based systems. Paper-based records are the predominant means of recording documentation. Many institutions are using or exploring methods of incorporating more computer-based documentation procedures. As facilities move from paper- to computer-based systems, it is not unusual for them to experience periods of time when portions of their procedures are paper-based, while other aspects are computer-driven.

Currently, paper-based systems are designed for data to be recorded in terms of the source of the information (such as therapy notes, or nurses' notes, or physician's notes), the time or timing of the information (daily or weekly notes), or the type of information (progress notes or discharge notes).

Paper-based documentation continues to dominate medical records based on a number of perceived advantages. They are considered to be:

- highly flexible and mobile
- easy to use, based on familiarity resulting from frequent usage
- complete, due to their complex, multiple-data format.

There are also distinct drawbacks to paper-based systems, such as:

- they are frequently seen as unreliable in that they are dependent upon the skill of the professional
- they are unavailable for multiple users at the same time
- illegibility frequently renders a note useless
- the time demands required to write a note may lead to shortcuts which eliminate important information.

Computer-based documentation, an alternative to the paper-based method, is increasing in popularity as computers become more commonplace. Once a computer system is set up, it becomes a simple and cost-effective means to document client data with increased ease and accuracy. There are numerous information management software systems on the market that allow the documentation of a wide range of client conditions accompanied by functional outcomes data. Most computer-based documentation systems are currently used in conjunction with paper-based systems. It is expected that computerized documentation will eventually emerge as the predominant method of recording data.

Current advantages of computerized documentation are:

1. Information can be easily accessed and updated.
2. There are fewer storage problems.
3. Information can be secured more easily.
4. It is easier to use recorded information to assess relationships among data.
5. There is increased consistency in format and style.

Drawbacks to computerized systems are expected to lessen as usage increases, but current disadvantages are perceived to be:

1. The capital investment for complete systems is extremely high.
2. Issues related to training staff and switching systems are frequently complex and troublesome.
3. The lack of compatibility among systems makes industry-wide connections almost impossible to achieve.

There is a problem-oriented method of recording that is commonly used in health care systems, in which information is recorded in terms of the presenting problems or the diagnosis. A commonly recognized form of problem-oriented documentation is referred to as the *SOAP* note format, in which client problems are listed and each member of the team writes a separate SOAP note to address the client's problem. SOAP is an acronym which allows for the following division of the patient record:

S = *S*ubjective
O = *O*bjective
A = *A*ssessment
P = *P*lan

Many facilities do not incorporate SOAP notes as a documentation technique. Other settings or specific disciplines within a setting have adapted the original SOAP format to one that is specifically geared to their needs. Whether SOAP notes are or are not incorporated into a intervention setting has not minimized the contribution they have made to organizing documentation approaches through their emphasis on the problem-oriented medical record (Kettenbach, 1990).

■ *Table 9.1.* **Sample of SOAP Note**

Subjective	Automatic speech echolalia
Objective	Seen to increase self-feeding and swallowing independence. Continues with restorative feeding and swallowing and ate 20% of meal. May try bolus feeding to facilitate return of appetite.
Assessment	Moderate assist for feeding is due to distractibility/fatigue and initiation apraxis. Moderate dysphagia with delayed swallow, manipulation of bolus posteriorly. Moderate increased tone in right elbow interferes with ability to bring food to mouth using dominant right upper extremity. Improvement continues with right labial closure (minimal spillage).
Plan	Continue self-feeding/swallow retraining. Consider orthosis to inhibit tone of right elbow.

Kettenbach, G. (1990), pp. 3–4. *Effective documentation for occupational therapy.* Philadelphia: F.A. Davis. Reprinted with permission.

Types of Notes

In addition to addressing the documentation delivery systems, documentation must also be explored in terms of the actual product of documentation, that is, the recorded note. Each note written by a practitioner has a specific purpose, and the practitioner must have a complete understanding of the purpose as the content of the note is developed. Several authors have categorized notes by purpose. Denton (1987) discusses the referral note, the initial note, the progress note, and the discharge note. Kettenbach (1990) describes initial notes, interim or progress notes, and discharge notes. In 1994, the American Occupational Therapy Association revised its description of clinical documentation, resulting in the categorization of documentation notes as:

1. the evaluation report (includes identification information, assessment results, and intervention or treatment plan)
2. the contact, treatment, or visit note
3. the progress report
4. the reevaluation report
5. the discharge or discontinuation report.

The content of each category is depicted in the following, which have been reprinted from the AOTA's *Elements of Clinical Documentation* (1994).

I. **Evaluation Report**—documents the initial contact with the consumer, the data collected, the interpretation of the data, and the intervention plan.

IA. **Identification and Background Information**

Content	Clarification
Name, age, sex, date of admission, treatment diagnosis, and date of onset of current diagnosis	Name may be omitted, depending on facility and department policies and procedures.
Referral source, services requested, and date of referral to occupational therapy	Who requested occupational therapy services, what specific services were requested, and date services were requested.
Medical history and secondary problems or preexisting conditions, prior therapy	Additional problems or conditions that may affect consumer functions or outcomes
Precautions and contraindications	May be identified by referral source or occupational therapy practitioners.
Pertinent history that indicates prior levels of function and support systems	Applicable developmental, educational, vocational, cultural, and socioeconomic history

Present levels of function in performance areas determined by examination	Brief description of the consumer's level of performance in activities of daily living, work and productive activities, and play or leisure activities
Performance contexts determined by examination	Description of those temporal aspects (chronological, developmental, life cycle, health status) and environmental (physical, social, cultural) features that affect the consumer's function in performance areas
Consumer and family expectations	Brief description of expected outcome of occupational therapy intervention

IB. Assessment Results

Content	Clarification
Tests and assessments administered and the results	Name and type of assessment or test and the results; may include comparison with the previous testing. State if standardized procedure followed.
References to other pertinent reports and information	Any additional sources of data or assessment results used
Summary and analysis of evaluation findings	State the type and severity of impairments identified and the functional limitations caused by the impairments in objective, functional, and measurable terms. Include the functional diagnosis.
Projected functional outcome(s)	Prognosis and anticipated level of performance (ADL, work or productive activities) the consumer will be able to achieve as a result of therapeutic intervention. May include a statement indicating that the consumer does not have the potential to improve beyond current status.

IC. Intervention or Treatment Plan

Content	Clarification
Long-term functional goals	Functional limitations that must change in order to achieve the projected functional outcome Degree the functional limitations will be decreased by x

	Rationale for decreasing functional limitations.
	Functional change to occur by end of x intervention
	Consumer and/or family agreement with goals
Short-term goals	Directly relate to long-term functional goals
	Impairment that must change in order to x achieve the projected functional outcome
	Degree the impairment will be decreased
	Functional ability that will result from an x decrease in level of impairment
	Change to occur in a brief period of time, e.g., 7, 14, or 30 days
	Consumer and/or family agreement with goals
Intervention or treatment procedures	Activities, techniques, and modalities selected to be used and how they relate to goals. May include family training and home programs. Identify assistive/adaptive equipment, orthotics, and/or prosthetics to meet consumer's environmental adaptation needs.
Type, amount, frequency, and duration of intervention or treatment	State skill and performance areas to be addressed and estimate the number, duration, and frequency of sessions to accomplish goals.
Recommendations	Need for occupational therapy services and necessary referrals to other professionals

II. Contact, Treatment, or Visit Note—used to document individual occupational therapy session or care coordination. May be very brief, such as in the use of a checklist, flow chart, or short narrative-type rotation.

Content	**Clarification**
Attendance and participation	Therapy occurrence or reason for therapy not occurring as scheduled

Activities, techniques, and modalities used	May be indicated by checklist or brief statement.
Assistive/adaptive equipment, prosthetics, and orthotics if issued or fabricated, and specific instructions for the application and/or use of the item.	State the device; note whether it was fabricated, sold, rented, or loaned; and state the effectiveness of the device.
Consumer's response to therapy	Level of performance and anything unusual or significant that was a result of occupational therapy intervention

III. Progress Report—used periodically to document care coordination, interventions, progress toward functional goals, and to update goals and intervention or treatment plan.

Content	Clarification
Activities, techniques, and modalities used	Brief statement of intervention process
Consumer's response to therapy, and the progress toward short- and long-term goal attainment and comparison with previous functional status	State the consumer's physical and behavioral response to therapy, whether the goals are being achieved, if change has occurred, and how much change has occurred.
Goal continuance	Explanation for no or slow progress, reason for not meeting short-term goals(s), or need to continue current goal(s)
Goal modification when indicated by the response to therapy or by the establishment of new consumer needs.	State new goals and rationale for changes or additions.
Change in anticipated time to achieve goals	If, for any reason, the therapy time frame is altered, include the reason for the change and the new anticipated time frame.
Assistive/adaptive equipment, prosthetics, orthotics, if issued or fabricated, and specific instructions for the application and/or use of the item	State the device; note whether it was fabricated, sold, rented, or loaned; and state the effectiveness of the device.
Consumer-related conferences and communication	If occupational therapy practitioners participated in a conference or made a pertinent contact with a faculty member, agency, or health care pro-

	fessional, state this information with a brief summary of the conference or communication.
Home programs	Include a copy of the home program as established with the consumer. Include a statement regarding the consumer's ability to follow the program.
Consumer/caretaker instructions	What instruction was provided and in what format (verbal or written)
Plan	Specific procedures, communication, or consultations to address future goals

IV. **Re-evaluation Report**—used to document sessions in which portions of the evaluation process are repeated or readministered. Usually occurs monthly or quarterly, depending on the setting.

Content	Clarification
Tests and assessments readministered	Name and type of test readministered. State if standardized procedure is not followed.
Comparative summary and analysis of previous findings	Results analyzed and compared with previous testing
Reestablishment of projected functional outcome(s)	Anticipated level of performance (ADL, work or productive activities, and play or leisure activities) the consumer will be able to achieve as a result of therapeutic intervention. May include a statement of changes in previously established functional outcome(s) based on revised potential or goals of consumer.
Update of intervention or treatment plan	Revised or continued long-term functional goals; short-term goals; treatment procedures; and type, amount, and frequency of therapy

V. **Discharge of Discontinuation Report**—used to document a summary of the course of therapy and any recommendations.

Content	Clarification
Therapy process	Summary of interventions used, consumer's responses, and number of sessions

Goal attainment	Degree to which short- and long-term, functional goals were achieved
Functional outcome	Comparison of functional status prior to therapy and at discharge
Home programs	Include the actual written home program that is to be followed after discharge.
Follow-up plans	State the schedule and specific plans.
Recommendations	State any recommendations pertaining to the consumer's future needs.
Referral(s) to other health care providers and community agencies	Indicate referral(s) or recommendations for referral(s) when additional or new services are needed.

The American Occupational Therapy Association. (1994). *Elements of clinical documentation.* Reprinted with permission.

As practitioners plan and write notes and plan the content of notes, it is critical that they remember that the notes are being written only from their professional perspectives as occupational therapy practitioners. The notes must relate to the meaning, goals, and underlying principles of occupational therapy. Notes written by an occupational therapy practitioner may address the same issues as notes written by other members of the team, but the practitioner's approach to the client and the problem, as described in the note, should reflect the concerns of occupational therapy, not nursing, not physical therapy, not social work, not any other profession. For the most part, every facility has its own unique approach to documentation and note writing. Within that format however, practitioners' notes include information related to data (results of screening, observations, interviews, performance assessments, evaluations); the interpretation of the data (problems and strengths); and a plan to affect the data (goals, objectives, methods); or, "the facts, what they mean, and what you plan to do about it" (Denton, 1987, p. 168).

Uniform Terminology for Occupational Therapy (3rd ed.) (Dunn, Foto, Hinojosa, Schell, Thompson, & Hertfelder, 1994) addresses *performance areas, performance components,* and *performance contexts.* These are the domains occupational therapy practitioners address during documentation and the writing of notes. By addressing functional performance and performance deficits in notes, therapists ensure the relevance of their notes to the true concerns of occupational therapy. It is not enough for practitioners to report data, as in degrees of flexion or minutes of endurance. Such information does not reflect the purposes of occupational therapy. Such data are meaningful only in the context of how they reflect performance. If, for example, the data related to flexion are linked to the patient's ability to dress or eat or swing a hammer, then this puts the information in a meaningful context of occupational therapy.

Maximizing Effective Documentation

Since "documentation of facts is the only evidence of professional decision-making" (Perinchief, 1993, p. 387), it is incumbent upon occupational therapy practitioners to convey documented information as clearly as possible. If written notes do not accurately communicate the intent of the practitioner, or if they are vague and ambiguous, leading to multiple interpretations by those who read them, then the notes have minimal effectiveness. Documentation requires a complicated set of skills. However, good, effective, and useable documentation can be learned and improved with practice. The goal of the practitioner is to record results of interactions so that others can read them, understand them, and recognize the importance of the contribution of occupational therapy to the intervention process.

One of the primary problematic areas for new practitioners is remembering that documentation is critical at each step in the other components of the intervention cycle. Less experienced practitioners frequently have difficulty recognizing that documentation makes the interview, the assessment, the observation, and the intervention plan complete. A note following each of these therapeutic interventions actually embeds them in reality. It communicates that something has indeed taken place. Without the record of events, the documentation of what occurred, it is as if nothing happened between the client and the practitioner.

Documentation is connected to intervention. As practitioners gain more skill and experience and increase their comfort with the intervention process, their ability to document effectively also improves. There are also certain language patterns that contribute to meaningful documentation. As practitioners understand the intervention process and their specific interventions, they acquire the language that is necessary for documentation. The more practitioners understand their interventions, the easier it is to document the results of treatment effectively.

Uniform Terminology (3rd ed.) (1994), the reporting system established by the Commission on Practice of the American Occupational Therapy Association, provides the basis for assuring that all documented information is understandable and transferable. Practitioners' familiarity with the *Uniform Terminology* can serve as a guiding factor in developing reports and writing notes. *Uniform Terminology* emphasizes occupational therapy's concern about functional performance, as it addresses the domains of performance areas, performance components, and performance contexts. Since performance is the realm of occupational therapy, it is expected that evaluation and assessment will focus on performance and performance deficits. If an occupational therapy intervention follows, it is expected to focus on maximizing performance and minimizing performance deficits. Effective, relevant, and occupation-based documentation will then relate the results of both the evaluation and intervention, in terms of performance. As a result of *Uniform Terminology*, practitioners from setting to setting are focused on the same concepts and use the same language. They can communicate with each other. Practitioners can document within the specific requirements of different facilities, while maintaining consistency and reflecting the essence of occupational therapy. By relying on *Uniform Terminology* as a documentation tool, practitioners are assured that their reports and notes are indicative of those professional perspectives that fall only within the purview of occupational therapy. Also important is that as practitioners increase their familiarity and comfort with *Uniform Terminology*, the frequency of use increases. The more *Uniform Terminology* is used in documentation, the more reimbursers and third-party payers understand the purposes and goals of occupational therapy. Increased understanding can then lead to a greater acceptance of occupational therapy services, as manifested by more trouble-free reimbursement practices.

Organizing and Planning Documentation Reports

Practitioners frequently encounter problems preparing good and effective notes. It may be helpful to consider the following points during the process of organizing and planning documentation reports.

CONSISTENCY

The importance of maintaining consistency between the multiple components of the intervention process cannot be stressed too strongly. The goals and intent of the evaluation and assessment, the speculations and conclusions of observations, the goals and results *must* reinforce each other as they relate to occupational therapy. Documentation then binds those components into a planned, integrated, and client-oriented regime. A frequent flaw in therapeutic interventions is for the therapist to evaluate using an assessment or methodology that reflects one frame of reference, develop goals and implement intervention based on another, and then write a note without mention of the results of either or without connecting them to the primary theme of the documentation. In addition to documentation being consistent with the other aspects of the program, component parts of the documentation must also be internally consistent, so that there are not contradictions within a note. For example, beginning a note with information about a client's positive attitude, but ending with a goal of improving the client's negative response to therapy, demonstrates inconsistency and will raise questions on the part of the reader.

BREVITY

Long, wordy notes are not read. The most effective documentation reports are those that are short and to the point. Documentation is not an exercise in creative writing but a reporting of fact. Extraneous information becomes a distraction. Florid embellishment raises questions about the validity of the content and can frequently lead to confusion and misinterpretation. In some settings, it is not required that full sentences be used; sentence fragments are acceptable and, in certain instances, preferred.

Some institutions or service delivery models have lists of acceptable abbreviations. The use of these abbreviations should be encouraged; however, the practitioner should note that while abbreviations may contribute to brevity, they may make a note incomprehensible to others. It is suggested that abbreviations be used with caution.

ACCURACY

The importance of accuracy is underscored when documentation is viewed as a legal, ethical, and financial record. Over time, memories fade regarding specific clients and associated interventions and interactions. If there is a need to review past occurrences, the documentation record is expected to be a reliable source. It is critical, therefore, that the record reflect information that is accurate and precise in every detail.

The following guidelines may help maximize accuracy of documentation.

General Guidelines

1. *Be certain that all handwritten documentation records are legibly written.* Handwritten notes can be meaningless if they cannot be read. Such notes are open to misinterpretation and may be completely ignored. At times, when a lengthy note is necessary, it is recommended that dictation be employed.
2. *Avoid forcing words into a line; avoid leaving blank spaces within an entry.* It can be difficult to read words that have been squeezed together; such words can be easily ignored or misinterpreted. Further, to avoid the possibility, however remote, of someone adding information to an already written note, it is best to draw a line through blank spaces after the end of an entry.
3. *Never erase, overwrite, or try to ink out any entry.* Of course, every attempt must be made to avoid mistakes, but, if one occurs, attempt to minimize ambiguity and confusion by drawing a *single* line through an incorrect entry with the date, time, and initials in the margin. Through such efforts, both the mistake

and the correction are clear. Such practices also reduce the risk of notes being altered by an unauthorized party.

4. *Never add anything to a previously entered record.* If a note is ever questioned, any alteration to a note, even if made by the original writer, can seriously compromise the integrity of the entire note. Additional information which the practitioner wants to include in the record should be transmitted in a separate, dated, and signed note.

5. *Avoid personal abbreviations.* Abbreviations should be kept to a minimum, but those that are included in a documentation record should be limited to the accepted abbreviations of the facility or service delivery model.

6. *Avoid lengthy, self-serving entries.* Wordy descriptions of occurrences may reflect information that is of interest to the practitioner but not relevant to the purpose of the documentation. Lengthy and subjective reporting may be dismissed as a defense mechanism of the practitioner.

It is important to emphasize that the above guidelines can contribute to accurate documentation, but true accuracy begins with the intervention process. The practitioner who understands the purposes of intervention, who plans and implements intervention based on the principles of occupational therapy, and who connects occupational therapy to the other aspects of intervention, is the practitioner who will more accurately document the record of the practitioner–client interaction. Accuracy in one segment of the treatment process is stimulated by accuracy in the other. This again exemplifies the importance of documentation in the intervention process and the interdependence of the component parts.

Documentation Writing Tips and Techniques

It would be most unfortunate for a therapist to effectively use highly refined observation and interview mechanisms, to select and utilize appropriate assessment techniques, to effectively evaluate performance and performance components, and to design an individualized intervention plan, and then have the meaning and effectiveness of this process lost, as a result of poorly-written documentation. A well-composed documentation report reveals what a practitioner knows about a client, as well as what is still to be determined. To communicate anything less is a disservice to the profession and to the recipient. The documentation note communicates the scope, range, and conclusions of therapy. If the note is written well, the reader receives a coherent picture of the occupational therapy services that were provided. If the note is not written well, it sometimes actually impedes the understanding of the note. The reader does not learn what the practitioner did, why it was done, or what was planned to be done in the future.

The following suggestions may be particularly helpful for the new practitioner with limited experience in documentation. It is true that more experience leads to more effective approaches to documenting. However, experienced practitioners must also be reminded of their writing style and its effect on documentation practices and results. The following writing tips are applicable to both paper-based and computer-based documentation methods.

1. *Maintain a "documentation" log.* Beginning practitioners frequently have negative feelings about documenting. Such feelings usually dissipate with experience, but one useful approach is to develop the habit of keeping a documentation log. The documentation log, similar to the learning log, is a private journal in which the practitioner can write freely about patient interactions, without being concerned about the conventions expected in formal documentation. Index cards or a small notebook can be used to jot down events, processes, reactions, and comments. Through such an exercise, a number of important synthesizing operations occur. The practitioner recreates, generalizes, and summarizes the intervention process, which serves to enrich understanding of not only what occurred, but of that which is relevant and important to communicate. Once such decisions are made, the practitioner can focus on the mechanics of recording the information.

2. *Organize information.* Although outlining is frequently viewed as a childish approach to writing, it actually has merit and can contribute to more-effective documentation. In the documentation log, the practitioner can arrange the information regarding interactions with the patient into clusters. Once information is clustered, it can then be sequenced. Which are most important and should be given first or saved for last? Which clusters must be present before others, in order to make key points understandable? These questions can be asked to determine the order of each cluster content; they can also assist in determining the sequence of content *within* each cluster. Through this process, the practitioner gains confidence about the logic and relevance of the documentation record's content.

3. *Start at the "right" point.* Before documenting, practitioners must determine how much is already known about the client. If this is not determined in advance, there is a possibility of documenting at too high or too low a level, which means reporting information that has already been recorded or eliminating information,

based on an assumption that it is recorded elsewhere. The practitioner must determine what has and has not been recorded and frame the documentation record to build on past content and prepare for future information.

4. *Avoid jargon.* Most practitioners spent many years learning the language of the profession. Professional language is indeed important; it frequently distinguishes one profession from another, and it is what communicates the essence of a given profession. It is no wonder that practitioners want to use their professional language as much as possible. Professional language is not problematic—when professionals talk among themselves. The problems occur when professional language dominates communication to other professional groups, such as through documentation processes. The best method is to simply avoid intraprofessional jargon, by using words that are common and familiar to all.

5. *Use "first-degree" words.* The concept of "first-degree" words may not be familiar. First-degree words immediately bring an image to mind. Second and third-degree words—some might call them "fifty-cent words"—must be translated through first-degree words before the image can be seen. First-degree words are always preferable.

First-degree words	Second/third-degree words
face	visage, countenance
stay	abide, remain, reside
book	volume, tome, publication

6. *Stick to the point.* The importance of using an outline (addressed in Point Two above) becomes evident at this stage. Any aspect of documentation can be assessed in terms of its relevance to the predeveloped outline. If the issue is referenced in the outline, more than likely it is relevant. If an issue is extraneous to the outline, it prompts the question: "Is this information off the track, or should it be added to the outline?"

7. *Avoid wordy phrases.* There is a tendency, even among experienced practitioners, to view words as means of "proving" to the outside world the importance of occupational therapy services. Such belief frequently leads to an excess verbiage that does not contribute to the understanding of a report.

Wordy phrases	Substitute
at the present time	now
in the event of	if
in the majority of circumstances	usually

In summary, the manner in which a documentation note is written can affect how it is received, assimilated, and utilized by the reader. Documentation serves as the confirmation that therapy actually occurred, and therefore it must be a well–written and easily-understood record of events. The writing tips listed above can help, but, nonetheless they remain only tips. We must strive to produce documentation reports that reflect integrated ideas that stem from a central theme and that support basic tenets of organization, flow, and cohesion of content.

Summary

Certainly, the ability to document effectively is not guaranteed by reading this chapter. Rather this chapter can be viewed as a beginning—one from which the practitioner can continue to build and develop documentation style and technique. The reader has been introduced here to the purposes and types of documentation, the importance of integrated documentation reports as they relate to the intervention process, and the methods of producing effectively presented reports. The application and incorporation of this content is up to each individual practitioner.

As with any skill, documentation requires practice and feedback in order to perfect it. Practitioners are encouraged to adapt documentation skills to the style of each practice arena in which they are working. They can adapt what has been learned to the development of a documentation style that is unique, individualized, and effective.

It is the responsibility of all occupational therapy practitioners to contribute to the development of the profession. By building documentation skills, every practitioner helps the profession move closer to a society-wide acceptance and understanding of the role of occupational therapy.

References

American Occupational Therapy Association. (1994). *Elements of clinical documentation.* Bethesda, MD: Author.

Denton, P.L. (1987). *Psychiatric occupational therapy: A workbook of practical skills.* Boston, Little, Brown.

Dunn, W., Foto, M., Hinojosa, J., Schell, B., Thompson, L.K., & Hertfelder, S.D., (1994). Uniform terminology for occupational therapy (3rd ed.). *American Journal of Occupational Therapy, 48,* 1039–1043.

Foto, M., Allen, C. Bass, C., Moon-Sperling, T., & Wilson, D. (1992). Reports that work. In J. Acquaviva (ed.), *Effective documentation for occupational therapy* (pp. 57–77). Bethesda. MD: American Occupational Therapy Association.

Kettenbach, G. (1990). *Writing S.O.A.P. notes.* Philadelphia: F.A. Davis.

Perinchief, J. (1993). Service management. In H. Hopkins & H. Smith (Eds.), *Willard and Spackman's occupational therapy* (pp. 375–398). Philadelphia: Lippincott.

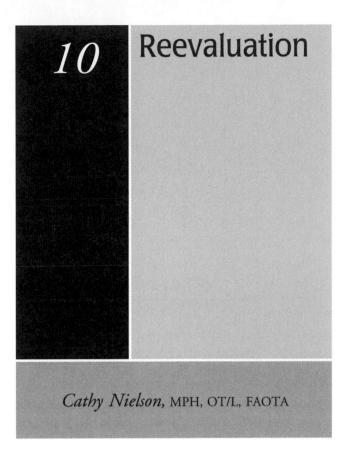

10 Reevaluation

Cathy Nielson, MPH, OT/L, FAOTA

Overview

This chapter introduces the process of reevaluation. It begins with information from American Occupational Therapy Association (AOTA) documents that reinforces the importance of reevaluation in the overall intervention process. The chapter presents reevaluation as a procedure parallel to initial evaluation that includes three steps: data collection, reflection, and decision-making. Included is a discussion of the forms of clinical reasoning that underlie and support each step in the reevaluation process. The chapter concludes with a brief overview of writing the reevaluation report.

Introduction

A variety of documents adopted by the AOTA underscore the need for occupational therapy practitioners to conduct ongoing or periodic reevaluation (AOTA, 1993; AOTA, 1994a; AOTA, 1994b; AOTA, 1995). In 1993, AOTA identified key performance areas for both occupational therapists and occupational therapy assistants. *Occupational Therapy Roles* (AOTA, 1993) lists monitoring the client's response to intervention, implementing modifications to the plan, and discontinuing intervention as key performance areas for the entry-level therapist. Similarly, key performance areas for the intermediate-level assistant include modifying intervention approaches in response to client needs and formulating discontinuation plans (both under the supervision of the occupational therapist). While the terms *reevaluation* and *reassessment* are not in the document, the ability to monitor the client and make modifications, including termination of services, is dependent upon the data collection, reflection, and decision-making steps of the reevaluation process.

The AOTA *Code of Ethics* (AOTA, 1994a) provides implicit support for reevaluation as a component of ethical practice. Principle 2.A. instructs occupational therapy practitioners to "collaborate with service recipients . . . in determining goals and priorities throughout the intervention process" (AOTA, 1994a, p. 1037), while Principle 3.D. directs personnel to use "accurate and current information" (AOTA, 1994a, p. 1037) as a basis for their performance. Inherent in these two principles is the notion that new information is continually introduced to the treatment process through systematic collection and analysis of client information, after the initial evaluation. Through Principle 4.A., the *Code of Ethics* mandates practitioners to follow applicable AOTA policies as well as laws, institutional policies, and procedures. Principle 3.B. advises adherence to the *Standards of Practice*, a document that explicitly establishes reevaluation as a professional standard.

The AOTA *Standards of Practice* (AOTA, 1994b) contains two standards that directly address reevaluation as a component of intervention. These standards follow.

> **Standard VI: Screening**
>
> A registered occupational therapist shall periodically reassess and document the individual's levels of functioning and changes in levels of functioning in the performance areas, performance components, and performance contexts.
>
> A certified occupational therapy assistant may contribute to the reassessment process under the supervision of a registered occupational therapist.
>
> A registered occupational therapist shall formulate and implement program modifications consistent with changes in the individual's response to the intervention. A certified occupational therapy assistant may contribute to program modification under the supervision of a registered occupational therapist (p. 1041).

These standards establish reevaluation as a minimum expectation in the provision of occupational therapy services.

A fourth AOTA document, *Elements of Clinical Documentation* (1995), presents information relative to reevaluation from the perspective of clinical documentation. The reevaluation report includes four content areas:

1. tests and assessments readministered and the results
2. comparative summary and analysis of previous evaluation findings
3. reestablishment of projected functional outcome(s)
4. update of intervention or treatment plan (p. 1034).

According to this document, the reevaluation report provides documentation of periodic reassessments that are readministered at intervals established by the practice setting.

The professional literature also contains multiple references supporting the concept that evaluation is continuous throughout the intervention or treatment process (Mattingly & Fleming, 1994; Muhlenhaupt, 1991; Opacich, 1991; Pelland, 1987; Pedretti, 1996; Trombly, 1995). Pedretti (1995) discusses reevaluation as occurring through both continuous observation and focused reassessment. The therapist considers the suitability of objectives from both the therapist's and client's perspectives and the appropriateness of methods, and modifies the plan based on analysis of that information.

Opacich (1991) effectively defends both the importance of reevaluation and its continuous nature in the following statement:

> But as we have seen, information-gathering and decision-making do not stop with the initial assessment and establishment of treatment goals. . . . data and clinical observations regarding changes in human performance are continuously collected in the course of therapy. The information serves to support, refute, or amend the treatment hypothesis and allows the clinician to make informed decisions. Furthermore, such evidence, systematically collected, can help determine the efficacy of treatment. If the therapy is not beneficial, the practitioner can decide to alter or terminate therapy. (p. 361)

Reevaluation, then, is simultaneous monitoring of the client and the effectiveness of the treatment plan, and a discrete activity involving the readministration of specific tests and procedures. Both types of reevaluation activities produce information used to modify the intervention approach.

A Three-Step Process

The occupational therapist initiates evaluation in order to determine the client's baseline status and to obtain information necessary for developing an intervention plan and intervention strategies. Reevaluation is a parallel process, producing information that enables the therapist to make modifications to the intervention plan and to continue to meet the changing needs of the client. Effective reevaluation is the integration of three steps: data collection,

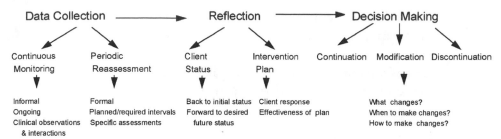

Figure 10.1. The Process of Reevaluation

reflection, and decision-making (Figure 10.1). Data collection includes both continuous and periodic components. The therapist then considers this information in terms of the client's changed status and the overall effect of the intervention or treatment plan. This leads to well-informed treatment decisions to modify, maintain, or discontinue discrete or comprehensive intervention strategies and actions.

STEP ONE—DATA COLLECTION

In the data collection step of reevaluation, the therapist gathers information about the client's current functional status relative to treatment goals, through both informal and formal methods. Informally, the therapist is continuously monitoring the client during each treatment session. The therapist collects and processes observations of the client's performance, verbal, nonverbal, and paraverbal responses to treatment activities. The clinician also integrates information from the caregiver or family member into the data base.

Through this continuous cycle of observation and interaction with the client and caregiver or family member, the therapist is able to introduce subtle and immediate changes in the intervention strategies. While the changes may appear to be intuitive, the therapist bases changes on observable clinical interactions and performance, and compares them retrospectively with the client's initial status and prospectively with the desired treatment outcome. When involved in the process of continuous monitoring, the therapist quickly merges the steps of data collection, reflection, and decision-making.

This ongoing approach to reevaluation is well-documented in the literature. Opacich (1991) refers to the process as "formative assessment" (p. 367). Muhlenhaupt (1991) writes of the need to evaluate a child's behavior as intervention progresses, comparing the new information to original performance and either making changes or maintaining the intervention plan. Continuous observation and assessment are discussed by Pedretti (1996) as a way of evaluating treatment effectiveness on an ongoing basis.

While continuous monitoring is an effective means of gathering evaluative information, the subjective nature of the data collection may limit its usefulness. There is also a need for planned periodic reassessment that includes objective methods of data collection. Periodic reassessment is a formal review of the client's status at a time designated within the initial intervention plan. This formal review may occur prior to writing a weekly progress note (Trombly, 1995) or at other regular intervals required by facility policy or reimbursement guidelines.

In this "summative" review (Opacich, 1991), the therapist reviews each problem area or critical area of function and compares each to the initial status and to the proposed goals. The therapist often readministers tests to gather objective evidence of change and validation of the intervention plan (Pedretti, 1996). The testing may be less extensive than at the time of initial assessment (Muhlenhaupt, 1991), as the reassessment focuses on discrete areas of problem or function. One consideration when using specific assessments in formal data collection is the test-retest reliability of the instrument. Therapists need to be familiar with the stability of the instrument over multiple administrations and the time intervals recommended for the instrument (Opacich, 1991). For a complete discussion of the implications of psychometrics in evaluation and assessment, the reader is referred to Chapter 5.

The dual processes of continuous monitoring and periodic reassessment result in a comprehensive clinical data base for the therapist's reflection and use in decision-making. Though either process can stand alone, ideally both should be done. The weaving together of the subjective and objective data provides a basis for the therapist to understand the client as an individual and to effectively evaluate both the client and the intervention plan.

STEP TWO—REFLECTION

The second step in reevaluation is reflection. In this step, the therapist considers all of the information obtained during formal and informal data collection. Initially, the therapist analyzes the information in terms of the client's status and identifies changes in the client's performance components, performance areas, or changes in the environment from the initiation of treatment or last reevaluation. Through this retrospective comparison, the therapist documents the progress, regression, or maintenance of the client's status. At the same time, the therapist reflects on the client's desired future state and evaluates how close the client is to that intervention outcome.

During the second component of the reflection step, the therapist evaluates the intervention plan. First, the therapist considers the client's response to the plan. The therapist again reflects on the changes in the client's performance components, areas, and environment, with an emphasis on identifying the aspects of the intervention plan that contributed to the change. The therapist must also consider more subjective information, including the client's reaction to and acceptance of intervention methods, the consistency of the client's objectives with the intervention objectives (Pedretti, 1996), and changes in the client's needs and desires.

This reflective process leads the therapist to a consideration of the overall effectiveness of the intervention plan. At this point, the therapist asks questions such as:

- Are the changes in the client's status meaningful to the individual or family?
- Are the changes important for functioning within his or her environment?
- Will the client, family, or caregiver be able to maintain these changes after discharge from therapy?
- Are the changes occurring at an appropriate rate and amount relative to the frequency and duration of treatment?
- How much more change can be expected?
- How much time is needed for the client to achieve the changes?

The therapist asks and answers questions like these, alone and in conjunction with the client, in order to move to decision-making, the final step of the reevaluation process.

STEP THREE—DECISION-MAKING

In this step of reevaluation, the therapist faces a choice of three decisions regarding the intervention plan: Continue the plan; modify the plan; or discontinue intervention and discharge the client from services. The therapist approaches the decision based on information gathered during step one and analyzed in step two. He or she thus arrives at the decision having considered all available information, and can provide a rationale for the decision.

The decision to continue the intervention without alteration indicates that the client is progressing satisfactorily and that the plan can continue to provide just the right challenge for achieving further progress. When the therapist decides to modify the intervention plan, he or she must also make subsequent decisions regarding the nature, timing, and implementation of the changes. The therapist may elect to adjust discrete treatment activities or approaches within the plan or may substantially alter the frequency, duration, and intensity of the entire plan.

Finally, the therapist can decide that it is time to discontinue treatment. Typically, the therapist makes this decision in one of several situations:

- when the client has achieved all intervention objectives and can sustain that progress outside of the treatment environment
- when the client is not able to meet all of the objectives but has achieved maximum therapeutic benefit
- when the client's personal needs, goals, or context changes.

When the therapist continues or modifies an intervention plan, then the therapist continues to cycle through the steps of data collection, reflection, and decision-making. The decision to terminate services ends the process of reevaluation.

Clinical Reasoning Through the Reevaluation Process

In their textbook on clinical reasoning, Mattingly and Fleming (1994) describe the process of clinical reasoning in occupational therapy as "deliberation about what an appropriate action is in this particular case, with this particular patient, at this particular time" (p. 10). They go on to describe procedural, interactive, and conditional reasoning (Mattingly & Fleming, 1994). Through these modes of reasoning, therapists learn the particulars of each case as the intervention plan is implemented and the relationship with the client unfolds.

Accordingly to this approach to clinical reasoning, therapeutic intervention begins in a biomedical mode, similar to medical diagnostic reasoning, as the therapist uses procedural reasoning to select and conduct initial assessments and to identify problems for intervention. As the treatment relationship develops, and the client and therapist get to know each other, the therapist shifts from procedural reasoning to interactive reasoning. Finally, the therapist moves to conditional reasoning, looking ahead to discharge and beginning to imagine the client's life after intervention. The process of reevaluation draws on all three reasoning modes.

As the therapist engages in continuous monitoring of the client, the primary mode of reasoning is interactive. Through numerous face-to-face encounters, the therapist and client share information about the intervention, how it feels, what it means, and what it will accomplish. As the relationship continues, the therapist learns more about the client's life and incorporates all of this information into refining the intervention plan. Once the decision is made to conduct a formal reassessment, the therapist switches into procedural reasoning, paralleling the thinking process of the initial assessment.

When reflecting on the client's status and the treatment plan, the therapist continues with procedural reasoning, as he or she identifies changes in the client's status and response to specific interventions. However, the therapist quickly shifts to interactive reasoning, as he or she reacts to subjective information from the client about his or her response to treatment, personal goals, and individual situation. A final shift to conditional reasoning occurs, as the therapist and client look ahead and compare the client's current status to the desired intervention outcome.

In decision-making, the final step in reevaluation, the therapist is again involved in multiple modes of reasoning. In continuing an existing intervention plan or selecting new intervention strategies, the therapist once more employs

■ *Table 10.1.* Primary Modes of Clinical Reasoning Associated with Steps of Reevaluation

Steps of Reevaluation	Primary Modes of Clinical Reasoning
Continuous monitoring	Interactive
Periodic reassessment	Procedural
Reflection on client status	Procedural, Conditional
Reflection on treatment plan	Interactive, Procedural
Decision-making	Procedural, Interactive, Conditional

Based on Mattingly, C. and Fleming M.H. (1994). *Clinical reasoning.* Philadelphia, PA: F.A. Davis.

procedural reasoning to match the plan and strategies to the problem or deficit. However, the therapist simultaneously moves to interactive reasoning, as the intervention plan is modified for the individual, and he or she is involved in decisions of how and when to modify the plan. When the therapist makes the decision to terminate services, a final switch to conditional reasoning occurs. The therapist and client again consider the client's life beyond the treatment setting and determine how able the client is to meet the demands and challenges of their life. Table 10.1. summarizes the primary modes of clinical reasoning associated with each step of the reevaluation process.

Mattingly and Fleming (1994) repeatedly reinforce the notion that reevaluation is an essential component of occupational therapy intervention. They identified "a process of nearly continuous hypothesis generation, evaluation, and revision" in occupational therapy (p. 336). This continuous process of revision is essential, no matter how thorough the initial assessment. The therapist, through reevaluation, is able to adjust the intervention to adapt to client improvement, regression, or evolution of the therapeutic relationship.

Other people have identified different methods of clinical reasoning. For a discussion of these reasoning processes, the reader is referred to Chapter 8.

Reevaluation Report

Once the process of reevaluation concludes, the therapist documents the results. The therapist can record reevaluation results, if brief, in the regular progress note, by recording the changes in client status and resulting adjustments in the intervention plan. Lengthy, comprehensive reports may require a separate format (Jabri, 1996). A comprehensive reevaluation report generally lists tests and assessments readministered, compares current and previous performance, reestablishes intervention outcomes, and updates the intervention plan (AOTA, 1995). Specific formats may be determined by the facility or the reimburser. The reader is referred to Chapter 9 for a complete discussion of documentation of a reevaluation.

Summary

Reevaluation is an essential component of the occupational therapy process. Through the steps of data collection, reflection, and decision-making, the therapist incorporates multiple pieces of information into a cohesive and responsive intervention plan. The data collection step includes continuous informal observations and interactions and planned use of specific assessments. The therapist reflects on the client's initial status and desired future status and considers the client's subjective responses in determining the effectiveness of the intervention plan. The therapist's evaluation of effectiveness leads to decisions about continuing, modifying, or discontinuing treatment. Through the three steps of reevaluation, the therapist is continually drawing on a blend of procedural, interactive, and conditional reasoning to make intervention decisions that are clinically sound, holistic, and responsive to the unique situation of the client.

References

American Occupational Therapy Association. (1993). Occupational therapy roles. *American Journal of Occupational Therapy, 47,* 1087–1099.

American Occupational Therapy Association. (1994a). Occupational therapy code of ethics. *American Journal of Occupational Therapy, 48,* 1037–1038.

American Occupational Therapy Association. (1994b). Standards of practice for occupational therapy. *American Journal of Occupational Therapy, 48,* 1039–1043.

American Occupational Therapy Association. (1995). Elements of clinical documentation (revised). *American Journal of Occupational Therapy, 49,* 1032–1035.

Jabri, J.L. (1996). Documentation of occupational therapy services. In L.W. Pedretti, *Occupational therapy practice skills for physical dysfunction* (4th ed.) (pp. 55–63). St. Louis, MO: Mosby.

Mattingly, C., & Fleming, M.H. (1994). *Clinical reasoning.* Philadelphia, PA: F.A. Davis.

Muhlenhaupt, M. (1991). Components of the program planning process. In W. Dunn (Ed.), *Pediatric occupational therapy,* pp. 125–138. Thorofare, NJ: Slack.

Opacich, K.J. (1991). Assessment and informed decision making. In C. Christiansen & C. Baum (Eds.), *Occupational therapy overcoming human performance deficits* (pp. 356–372). Thorofare, NJ: Slack.

Pedretti, L.W. (1996). Treatment planning. In L.W. Pedretti, *Occupational therapy practice skills for physical dysfunction* (4th ed.) (pp. 46–54). St. Louis, MO: Mosby.

Pelland, M.J. (1987). A conceptual model for the instruction and supervision of treatment planning. *American Journal of Occupational Therapy, 41,* 351–359.

Trombly, C.A. (1995). Planning, guiding and documenting therapy. In C.A. Trombly (Ed.), *Occupational therapy for physical dysfunction* (pp. 29–40). Baltimore: Williams & Wilkins.

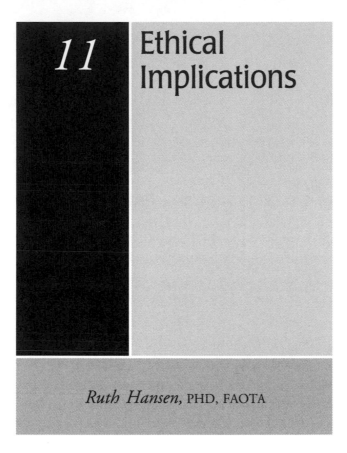

11 Ethical Implications

Ruth Hansen, PHD, FAOTA

Overview

The primary purpose of this chapter is to discuss the ethical parameters of assessment. The chapter begins with a discussion of personal and professional values. The reader will have the opportunity to consider his or her own personal values and determine how they coincide with or differ from the profession's values. Next is a section that describes some of the ethical issues to consider when conducting assessments. Finally, the reader will learn how to identify and analyze ethical dilemmas that arise in this process.

Introduction

In her 1983 Eleanor Clarke Slagle lecture, Joan Rogers described the science, the art, and the ethics of clinical reasoning. She posed questions to answer at each step in the intervention process: What is the patient's status? (science); what are the available options? (art); and what ought to be done? (ethics) (Rogers, 1983). Rogers placed more emphasis on the ethics of clinical reasoning in the planning and implementation portions of the therapeutic process. Nonetheless, ethical considerations are equally important in the assessment phase of the process.

Decisions about what is the correct action in a given situation are part of our daily lives. We make those determinations of right or wrong based on our personal and professional values. Ethical dilemmas exist because there are no clear-cut answers in many practice situations. There may be two or more options. However, in most cases, it has been found that there is a single, best solution (Hansen, 1990).

Origins of Personal and Professional Values

We base our practice decisions on a combination of our personal beliefs and values, and the values that the occupational therapy profession espouses.

Our personal values evolve from our individual experiences and interactions. Some of the key factors that contribute to the formation of our values are:

- our religious, spiritual or personal beliefs about right and wrong
- our family traditions, standards, and interactions
- our culture and the norms of the society in which we live
- the influence of friends, colleagues, and teachers
- the writings and speeches of individuals who are important or influential in our lives.

Personal values evolve and change over a lifetime of experiences. According to Kohlberg, Gilligan, Perry, and other moral development theorists (Kurtines & Gewirtz, 1991), our stage of moral development or moral reasoning determines to some extent how we make moral decisions. Along with the variables listed above, changes in the individual's general intelligence, information-processing skills, educational level, and socialization can change the person's level of moral reasoning (Kay, 1982). In earlier studies, James Rest (1979) found that the person's level of education was more predictive of the level of moral reasoning than age. "Cognitive restructuring of one's moral thinking seems to be more related to years in school than to years since birth in adults" (p. 73).

It is important that we know and understand our own values and have a clear picture of what we believe to be right and wrong. However, even with a clear set of personal standards or values, deciding what is the best solution under specific circumstances will not be simple.

Professional values. What are they? Where do they come from? The occupational therapy profession has developed several official statements that describe the professional values important to us. These statements are developed by the consensus of the whole profession. This consensus is achieved through discussion and deliberation. There is also an aspect of our professional values that exists because of the nature of the work we do and the similarities between that work and the inherent values one must hold to perform that work. Individuals are attracted to occupational therapy to some extent because of the harmony between their personal values and the values of the profession. ("I value independence and helping others to achieve independence. Concomitantly, occupational therapy values independence and providing people with the means to achieve their goals.")

The formation and acceptance of professional values is facilitated by formal education and close association with professional colleagues. We are socialized to the values of our profession by our teachers, classmates, supervisors, team members, and professional mentors. If an admired colleague or professor values each individual as a unique human being and behaves in ways that enforce that belief, you may find that you have assumed the same value or have placed it as a higher priority in your own value system. The ideal result for a member of the profession is that there is harmony between personal and professional values.

There are two key documents of the American Occupational Therapy Association that describe our professional values. The first is the *Occupational Therapy Code of Ethics* (AOTA, 1994) (Appendix D), and the second is the *Core Values and Attitudes of Occupational Therapy Practice* (Kanny, 1993).

These documents have some similarities. The code contains six principles that describe the values and behaviors to which members of the profession should aspire. The main ideas included in this document are:

- beneficence, or the importance of doing good for others
- nonmaleficence, or the need to avoid doing harm
- respecting the rights of individuals to autonomy, privacy, and confidentiality
- the need to know and abide by the laws and regulations that govern practice
- the duty to maintain and promote high standards of competence, including the exercise of sound clinical judgment
- the need to be truthful (veracity) in providing accurate information to those receiving our services, as well as charging reasonable fees for those service
- the importance of treating our professional colleagues with fairness, discretion, and integrity.

Core Value and Attitudes in Occupational Therapy Practice describes the beliefs that have served as an underpinning for the profession since its inception. There are seven core concepts identified:

1. Altruism, or concern for the welfare of others
2. Equality, or the belief that all individuals have the same fundamental human rights and opportunities

3. Freedom to exercise choice and be independent
4. Justice, or the importance of upholding the moral and legal principles of fairness, equity, truthfulness, and objectivity
5. Dignity, emphasizing the importance of valuing the inherent worth and uniqueness of each person
6. Truth, or being faithful to the facts and reality
7. Prudence, or the ability to govern and discipline oneself through reasoning.

Certainly these two documents have similar themes: doing good for others, treating individuals with fairness and equity, being truthful, and upholding high standards of professional conduct and competence. They are different in the emphasis and language used to describe the key concepts because they were written for different purposes. *Core Values and Attitudes in Occupational Therapy Practice* is a retrospective description of the values and attitudes that have prevailed in our profession. The author examined core documents of the profession to determine what the prevailing values and attitudes are. *Occupational Therapy Code of Ethics*, on the other hand, is a statement that assures the public that members will conduct themselves in a manner above that expected of other citizens. Society allows professionals certain privileges. We have access to confidential information about individuals, and we have permission to touch and manipulate another person's body in the process of carrying out therapy. The Code is our pledge to hold ourselves to a higher standard and to protect the rights of the people that seek our services.

■ *Figure 11.1.*   Core Values and Attitudes of Occupational Therapy Practice

Introduction

In 1985, the American Occupational Therapy Association (AOTA) funded the Professional and Technical Role Analysis Study (PATRA). This study had two purposes: to delineate the entry-level practice of OTRs and COTAs through a role analysis and to conduct a task inventory of what practitioners actually do. Knowledge, skills, and attitude statements were to be developed to provide a basis for the role analysis. The PATRA study completed the knowledge and skills statements. The Executive Board subsequently charged the Standards and Ethics Commission (SEC) to develop a statement that would describe the attitudes and values that undergird the profession of occupational therapy. The SEC wrote this document for use by AOTA members.

The list of terms used in this statement was originally constructed by the American Association of Colleges of Nursing (AACN) (1986). The PATRA committee analyzed the knowledge statements that the committee had written and selected those terms from the AACN list that best identified the values and attitudes of our profession. This list of terms was then forwarded to SEC by the PATRA Committee to use as the basis for the Core Values and Attitudes paper.

The development of this document is predicated on the assumption that the values of occupational therapy are evident in the official documents of the American Occupational Therapy Association. The official documents that were examined are: (a) *Dictionary Definition of Occupational Therapy* (AOTA, 1986), (b) *The Philosophical Base of Occupational Therapy* (AOTA, 1979), (c) *Essentials and Guidelines for an Accredited Educational Program for the Occupational Therapist* (AOTA, 1991a), (d) *Essentials and*

---

continued

■ *Figure 11.1.* continued

Guidelines for an Accredited Educational Program for the Occupational Therapy Assistant (AOTA, 1991b), and (e) *Occupational Therapy Code of Ethics* (AOTA, 1988). It is further assured that these documents are representative of the values and beliefs reflected in other occupational therapy literature.

A *value* is defined as a belief or an ideal to which an individual is committed. Values are an important part of the base or foundation of a profession. Ideally, these values are embraced by all members of the profession and are reflected in the members' interactions with those persons receiving services, colleagues, and the society at large. Values have a central role in a profession and are developed and reinforced throughout an individual's life as a student and as a professional.

Actions and attitudes reflect the values of the individual. An attitude is the disposition to respond positively or negatively toward an object, person, concept, or situation. Thus, there is an assumption that all professional actions and interactions are rooted in certain core values and beliefs.

Seven Core Concepts

In this document, the *core values and attitudes* of occupational therapy are organized around seven basic concepts—altruism, equality, freedom, justice, dignity, truth, and prudence. How these core values and attitudes are expressed and implemented by occupational therapy practitioners may vary depending upon the environments and situations in which professional activity occurs.

Altruism is the unselfish concern for the welfare of others. This concept is reflected in actions and attitudes of commitment, caring, dedication, responsiveness, and understanding.

Equality requires that all individuals be perceived as having the same fundamental human rights and opportunities. This value is demonstrated by an attitude of fairness and impartiality. We believe that we should respect all individuals, keeping in mind that they may have values, beliefs, or life-styles that are different from our own. Equality is practiced in the broad professional arena, but is particularly important in day-to-day interactions with those individuals receiving occupational therapy services.

Freedom allows the individual to exercise choice and to demonstrate independence, initiative, and self-direction. There is a need for all individuals to find a balance between autonomy and societal membership that is reflected in the choice of various patterns of interdependence with the human and nonhuman environment. We believe that individuals are internally and externally motivated toward action in a continuous process of adaptation throughout the life span. Purposeful activity plays a major role in developing and exercising self-direction, initiative, interdependence, and relatedness to the world. Activities verify the individual's ability to adapt, and they establish a satisfying balance between autonomy and societal membership. As professionals, we affirm the freedom of choice for each individual to pursue goals that have personal and social meaning.

Justice places value on the upholding of such moral and legal principles as fairness, equity, truthfulness, and objectivity. This means we aspire to provide occupational therapy services for all individuals who are in need of these services and that we will maintain a goal-directed and objective relationship with all those served. Practitioners must be knowledgeable about and have respect for the legal rights of individuals receiving occupational therapy services. In addition, the occupational therapy practitioner must understand and abide by the local, state, and federal laws governing professional practice.

Dignity emphasizes the importance of valuing the inherent worth and uniqueness of each person. This value is demonstrated by an attitude of empathy and respect for self and others. We believe that each individual is a unique combination of biologic endowment, sociocultural heritage, and life experiences. We view human beings holistically, respecting the unique interaction of the mind, body, and physical and social environment. We believe that dignity is nurtured and grows from the sense of competence and self-worth that is integrally linked to the person's ability to perform valued and relevant activities. In occupational therapy we emphasize the importance of dignity by helping the individual build on his or her unique attributes and resources.

continued

■ *Figure 11.1.* continued

Truth requires that we be faithful to facts and reality. Truthfulness or veracity is demonstrated by being accountable, honest, forthright, accurate, and authentic in our attitudes and actions. There is an obligation to be truthful with ourselves, those who receive services, colleagues, and society. One way that this is exhibited is through maintaining and upgrading professional competence. This happens, in part, through an unfaltering commitment to inquiry and learning, to self-understanding, and to the development of an interpersonal competence.

Prudence is the ability to govern and discipline oneself through the use of reason. To be prudent is to value judiciousness, discretion, vigilance, moderation, care, and circumspection in the management of one's affairs, to temper extremes, make judgments, and respond on the basis of intelligent reflection and rational thought.

Summary

Beliefs and values are those intrinsic concepts that underlie the core of the profession and the professional interactions of each practitioner. These values describe the profession's philosophy and provide the basis for defining purpose. The emphasis or priority that is given to each value may change as one's professional career evolves and as the unique characteristics of a situation unfold. This evolution of values is developmental in nature. Although we have basic values that cannot be violated, the degree to which certain values will take priority at a given time is influenced by the specifics of a situation and the environment in which it occurs. In one instance dignity may be a higher priority than truth; in another prudence may be chosen over freedom. As we process information and make decisions, the weight of the values that we hold may change. The practitioner faces dilemmas because of conflicting values and is required to engage in thoughtful deliberation to determine where the priority lies in a given situation.

The challenge for us all is to know our values, be able to make reasoned choices in situations of conflict, and be able to clearly articulate and defend our choices. At the same time, it is important that all members of the profession be committed to a set of common values. This mutual commitment to a set of beliefs and principles that govern our practice can provide a basis for clarifying expectations between the recipient and the provider of services. Shared values empowers the profession and, in addition, builds trust among ourselves and with others.

References

American Association of Colleges of Nursing (1986). *Essentials of College and University Education for Professional Nursing, Final report.* Washington, DC: Author.

American Occupational Therapy Association. (1979). The philosophical base of occupational therapy. *American Journal of Occupational Therapy, 33,* 785.

American Occupational Therapy Association. (1986, April). *Dictionary definition of occupational therapy.* Adopted and approved by the Representative Assembly to fulfill Resolution #596-83. (Available from AOTA, 4720 Montgomery Lane, PO Box 31220, Bethesda, MD 20824.)

American Occupational Therapy Association. (1988). Occupational therapy code of ethics. *American Journal of Occupational Therapy, 42,* 795–796.

American Occupational Therapy Association. (1991a). Essentials and guidelines for an accredited educational program for the occupational therapist. *American Journal of Occupational Therapy, 45,* 1077–1084.

American Occupational Therapy Association. (1991b). Essentials and guidelines for an accredited educational program for the occupational therapist. *American Journal of Occupational Therapy, 45,* 1085–1092.

Prepared by Elizabeth Kanny, MA, OTR, for the Standards and Ethics Commission (Ruth A. Hansen, PhD, OTR, FAOTA, Chairperson). Approved by the Representative Assembly June 1993.

Source: *The American Journal of Occupational Therapy,* 47, December 1993, 1085–1086.

Ethical Considerations in Assessment

The key concepts in the two professional documents discussed above can be the basis for an examination of some specific ethical issues regarding assessment. The first step is to consider the multiple forces and types of interests that make up the context in which an assessment is taking place. To whom does the practitioner have a primary duty when making decisions about what evaluations to used, how to report the data, and to whom the data should be reported? Most of us think of the client or consumer as our first priority. There are also the family and significant others, our employer and the facility for which we work, our fellow professionals, and the agency or individual who is paying for the assessment. It should be easy to see how conflicts can arise as the priorities, goals, and values of the different individuals and groups clash or, at least, do not coincide.

When the client is of the age of maturity as defined by state regulations and is able to make his or her own decisions, the practitioner's first responsibility is to that client. This means that data or evaluation results cannot be released to family members, significant others, or professionals without consent. When a client is a minor or not able to make his or her own decisions, the responsibility for consent to release information is held by the parent or legal guardian. During the evaluation process, a practitioner may discover information or observe physical evidence that bears upon the client's safety. In such cases, where abuse or neglect is suspected, the practitioner has the ethical and moral responsibility to inform state authorities, in concert with state law, in order to protect the client. While it may be helpful to discuss this situation with the legal guardian, this may not always be possible. The practitioner has the responsibility to report such suspicions.

The key issue is a thorough examination of the concerns, rights, duties, and vested interests of each player in a given situation (Hansen, 1990). Table 11.1 is a list of some of the key questions that the practitioner should ask when reviewing the ethical (and legal) issues involved in the evaluation and assessment process.

Each of the players described in Table 11.1 has a different role to play in the assessment process. The following paragraphs provide some explanations of how ethical conflicts may arise and why the questions that are posed have ethical importance.

Occupational therapists should ask, "Am I competent to do this assessment?" Therapists are legally and ethically bound to be sure they are competent to engage in all aspects of their practice. They must have the knowledge, skills, and attitudes to select, administer, and interpret the results of each evaluation.

They should ask themselves, "Am I competent to supervise other occupational therapy personnel in the collection of data for this assessment?" Thera-

■ *Table 11.1.* **Questionnaire for Identifying Potential Conflicts**

Occupational Therapist
- Am I competent to do this assessment? Do I have the necessary knowledge, skills, and attitudes to select, administer, and interpret the results of each evaluation?
- Am I competent to supervise other occupational therapy personnel in the collection of data for this assessment? Am I sure that all delegated tasks are being carried out properly by competent individuals?
- Have I accurately documented the services provided? Is the summary assessment an accurate reflection of the separate evaluations?

Occupational Therapy Assistant
- Am I competent to carry out the data collection that I am responsible to perform?
- Am I receiving adequate training and supervision to carry out the assigned portions of the assessment process?
- Have I accurately reported the data and contributed to the overall assessment process?

Individual who is being assessed (family, significant others, guardian)
- Has the consumer been informed about the purpose of the assessment, how it will be administered, and by whom? Does this person understand how the results of the assessment will be used?
- Has the individual been informed about how this service will be billed?
- Has the person been given the opportunity to decide if the assessment should be done?
- Are the individual's goals the basis for developing and carrying out the assessment process?

Employer (facility, agency, company)
- Is the assessment consistent with the mission of the facility?
- Will there be an accurate billing for services?
- How will the interpretation and recommendations of the therapist be used?

Payer
- Is the assessment a necessary and billable service?
- If there is not coverage by third-party reimbursement, does the client know this? Has this individual given consent before the initiation of the evaluations?
- Will the therapist and the billing office request fair compensation for the services and request payment only for the services provided?

Professional colleagues
- Is the referral consistent with the client's goals and needs?
- Is this assessment necessary?
- Are you communicating the results of the assessment clearly so that other members of the service delivery team have useful information?
- Have copyrighted evaluation materials been used according to the laws regulating their use?
- Is it necessary to pay fees to use the evaluation tool? Have they been paid?
- Must the practitioner obtain permission to use the materials?
- Is there specific training and supervision required to conduct the evaluation?
- Does the person carrying out the evaluation hold the appropriate credentials to do so?
- Have you used the correct forms and procedures in conducting the evaluation and reporting the results?
- If it is a standardized evaluation, have you followed the procedures exactly?

Community and society
- Is this assessment consistent with the concepts of due process, reparation for wrongs that have been done (physical or emotional), and the fair and equitable distribution of occupational therapy services to individuals needing those services?

Revised from Hansen, R.A. (1990). Lesson 10: Ethical considerations. In C.B. Royeen (Ed.), *AOTA Self study series. Assessing functions* (p. 9). Bethesda, MD: American Occupational Therapy Association.

pists must also be sure that they are capable of providing adequate supervision if they choose to delegate any portion of the assessment process to other personnel. The responsibility for assuring that delegated tasks are being carried out properly by competent individuals rests with the supervisor.

"Have I accurately documented the services provided?" Occupational therapists must have the ability to document the assessments included in the final evaluation in a manner that is both valid and reliable. Being able to summarize information from multiple sources in an overall assessment of the person's function is both a complex and a crucial process for the person being evaluated. Therapists must be certain that the evaluation accurately reflects the information from the individual assessments.

"Am I using language that is respectful of the autonomy and integrity of the individual receiving the assessment?" Careful selection of terms used to describe the function of the individual is important for legal, fiscal, and ethical reasons. Selecting words that others may use to label a person can cause irreversible damage to the autonomy and integrity of the individual. For example, during one observation, a therapist notes that a person is unable to concentrate on a paper and pencil task for more than 3 minutes, is unable to sit in a chair for more than 5 minutes, and is distracted by people and noises outside the room. There are choices about how this information is reported. If the therapist uses language such as "hyperactive," or "attention deficit disorder," the individual may be stigmatized unnecessarily. For a child, this may have a significant impact on his or her educational program, which may not be in the child's best interest. Professionals need to be very sensitive to the use of "labels" to categorize the function or behaviors of an individual as a particular syndrome, condition, or diagnosis.

Another aspect of written and verbal language that indicates respect of the individual is to refrain from referring to an individual by the diagnosis. Do not refer to a person as "a quad," "an amputee," "the anorexic," "the schizophrenic." It is also insensitive to refer to the "mentally retarded child," the "stroke patient," the "cerebral palsied kid." Although such shorthand language is commonplace in clinics and medical records, it negates the individuality of the person. Each of us is a person, with a variety of traits that can be used to describe aspects of our personality, behavior, and function. To use a disease or condition as the adjective preceding the identifying noun negates the multiple dimensions that make the person a unique individual.

Occupational therapy assistants must also be sure that they are competent to carry out the date collection procedures they are responsible to complete. They must receive adequate training to carry out assigned tasks and must have adequate supervision throughout this process.

The occupational therapy assistant needs to provide accurate and clear documentation when contributing data. Occupational therapy assistants must also take the same degree of care in selecting language that avoids labeling the person and that puts the person first in the description of observed dysfunction.

The next important player is the *consumer*—the individual who is being assessed, as well as that person's family and significant others. Personnel who are administering assessments must make every attempt to ensure that the consumer knows and understands the purpose of the assessment, how the portions of it will be administered, and who will administer each portion. The consumer also needs to know how the results of the assessment will be used in the process of making determinations about future services, types of care, placement, etc.

It is important to make sure that the consumer knows and understands what the assessment will cost and how it will be paid for. When the assessor is reasonably certain that the consumer is fully informed, the next step is to give the consumer the opportunity to accept or refuse the assessment.

Also, the planning and implementation of the evaluation process must be congruent with the consumer's interests and goals. At the completion of the evaluation, the final recommendation and goals must be congruent with those that the consumer has identified. The consumer must be given the opportunity to acknowledge that these goals are both acceptable and desirable.

The *employer* also has an important role in the assessment process. Whether the assessor is self-employed or works for someone else, the mission of agency or organization will influence what services are provided, when they are provided, and where they are provided. The facility also has influence over who will perform various evaluations and the purposes for which the information is being gathered. The person carrying out the assessment must understand all of the factors and be comfortable providing assessments within that framework.

The next question is, will there be accurate billing for the services provided? The therapist must know the billing practices used in the facility and determine that the charges are both reasonable and fair.

The therapist must understand how the results of an assessment will be interpreted and used. Earlier I mentioned the need for care in the use of language when writing an evaluation. Similarly, there needs to be a clear understanding of how the evaluation results will be used by others, as well as who will make the recommendations and how they will be carried out.

Another important part of evaluation is taking into consideration who is paying for these services. The payer will want to know if the assessment is a necessary and billable service. The therapist needs to know whether the services that will be provided will be covered by third-party reimbursement. Does the consumer have third-party coverage? Will that provider pay for the assessment? In cases where the consumer does not have third-party coverage, the therapist must inform the individual what the assessment will cost. The consumer will have to provide approval and consent before the initiation of the assessment.

It is also incumbent upon the therapist to make sure that the employer is requesting fair compensation for the services provided and that the billing office is requesting payment only for those services provided.

In the evaluation process, it is necessary and important to interact with various *professional colleagues*. In this process, additional questions arise. Is the referral for assessment consistent with the consumer's goals and needs? Is this assessment necessary? It is also essential to communicate the results of an assessment in language that is understood by everyone on the "team," including the consumer. If highly technical terms or jargon are used, the results of the evaluation will, at best, not be clear and, at worst, will be misconstrued.

Another point related to professional colleagues is to be sure that any copyrighted materials are used in accordance with the laws that regulate their use. The therapist should know whether any evaluations that are being used are copyrighted. If so, then the questions that come to mind are: Are there fees that must be paid to use this evaluation? If so, have those fees been paid? It is illegal to photocopy copyrighted materials and use them. Is it necessary to obtain permission to use the evaluation materials? Some evaluations are available without charge but may require that permission be obtained from the author. Are training and supervision required to conduct the evaluation? For example, the Sensory Integration and Praxis Tests should not be used unless the assessor has been certified by Sensory Integration International. Does the person doing the evaluation hold the appropriate credentials to do this evaluation? Some evaluations, like the Vineland Adaptive Behavior Scales (Sparrow, Balla & Circhetti, 1984), indicate that the evaluator should be a licensed psychologist. Also, the therapist must be sure to use the correct forms and procedures when conducting the evaluation and when reporting the results. If the evaluation is standardized, then the procedures for doing the evaluation must be carried out as stipulated in the test manual.

Many of the evaluations that are used by practitioners are not copyrighted. If the evaluation has been developed by someone else, that individual should be properly acknowledged when the evaluation is used. Otherwise the assumption will be made that the evaluation is original to the practitioner who is doing the evaluation. This is rarely the case.

The other constituent group that needs to be taken into consideration is the *community* or *society at large*. Here, the therapist must be attuned to the procedures for due process. Due process is the prescribed course of action to protect the legal rights of individuals. For example, if the results of an evaluation may be used to determine whether the person is placed in a specific facility, that person's interest must be fairly and equitably considered. There are also implications when the consumer is receiving an evaluation in order to determine the amount and type of compensation to be received for wrongs (either physical or emotional). Finally, the issue of access to appropriate personnel and assessment is vital. Decisions about who receives care are often made by gatekeepers, the people who control access to the system or service. As a result, there is concern about whether there is fair and equitable distribution of occupational therapy services to individuals who need those services.

You can use this list of questions to remind yourself of the various ethical dimensions included in the evaluation process. In this list, several themes reoccur. One is related to documentation. Who will pay for the services? How many others use the results? Has the evaluation been requested as a means of initiating treatment? If so, are there limitations on the type of therapy that can be provided? Will the results be used to determine the individual's level of competence; to select appropriate placement; to substantiate the person's degree of function or dysfunction? Will the results be used to determine whether to initiate, continue, alter, or curtail compensation for disability? Will the results be used as evidence in pending litigation?

Linked to the questions of who will pay for the evaluation and the purpose of the evaluation is the need to determine whether the consumer has been informed. The practitioner must be sure that the client receives this information and has the opportunity to accept or refuse the evaluation. When clients are unable to make their own decisions, practitioners must make sure that those people responsible for the client are likewise informed. Informed consent is problematic when it is unclear whether the individual can act in his or her own best interests. Informed consent can also be compromised when the results of the evaluation are tied to disability compensation or financial restitution for damages (Hansen, 1990).

System for the Analysis of Ethical Dilemmas

Another useful tool when dealing with ethical issues related to evaluation is a systematic method of analysis. This system can help to resolve evaluation dilemmas. Many ethicists suggest strategies to use for identifying and prioritizing the salient issues of a conflict. The method described in this chapter was developed by Hansen, Kyler-Hutchison, and Trompetter (1994), based on the work of Aroskar (1980).

As Table 11.2 shows, this system consists of another series of focused questions that the occupational therapist answers in order to weigh possible solutions and their consequences. The outcome is a resolution that is clear, explainable, and defensible.

The case analysis that follows will give an idea of how this process works. This analysis was written by Sharon "Maggie" Reitz for an article that I co-authored with her and Linda Kamp in the May 1988 issue of the *American Journal of Occupational Therapy.*

■ *Table 11.2.* System of Ethical Analysis

1. Who are the players in the dilemma?
2. What other facts/information do you need?
3. What are the actions that might be taken?
4. What are the consequences (ethical and legal) of each action?
5. Choose an action or combination of actions that you would recommend and defend it.
   - Is it legal?
   - Is it balanced? Fair to all concerned?
   - Does it set up a win-win situation, if possible?
   - How does the decision make you feel about yourself?

From Hansen, R.A., Kyler-Hutchison P.L., & Trompetter, L. (1994). Ethical issues and the health professions. *1994 Special Lecture Series.* College Misericordia, Occupational Therapy Program, Dallas, PA.

Case Example

An occupational therapist is working in a day care facility with clients who have developmental disabilities. The goal in providing these services at this site is to serve clients in the least restrictive environment available. All clients are screened prior to consideration for admission.

Recently, a client was screened for admission. The occupational therapist determined that the client was functioning at a relatively high level. The therapist did not feel that this person required the services of the facility but that placement should be in a less restrictive environment, provided by another agency. Nonetheless, the owners of the facility wanted to admit this client because the current census is low. In fact, in order to provide for higher occupancy and greater revenue, the client was admitted to the center, contrary to the recommendations of the occupational therapist.

At this point, the occupational therapist is torn between the conviction of a well–established and documented professional judgment and a need to be loyal to and supportive of the owners of the facility.

What should the therapist do and why? ■

Additional information/facts. The therapist should first gather any pertinent facts in order to answer the following three questions:

1. Is the client competent to choose a facility? If not, did the family select the facility? Has the decision-making party been informed of the OT evaluation/recommendations?
2. Is there a conveniently located higher-level facility/program that the family can afford?

3. Are there other reasons, such as family wishes, that the owners also took into consideration when choosing to admit the client?

Alternative actions.

1. Quit in protest.
2. Request a meeting with the owners and present the ethical dilemma they are facing (client's needs versus employer's needs) and seek to resolve the issue.
3. Meet with the family members and provide them with the information that the therapist used to come up with the recommendations about the client's placement.
4. Do nothing and ignore the situation, rationalizing that it's the owners' responsibility, and they have to live with the decision.

To assist you in resolving the dilemma presented by this case, see Table 11.3.

Weighing the issues and recommended action. Obviously, actions 1 and 4 are unacceptable. Actions 2 and 3 are related and are dependent on the outcome of one another. The therapist should first approach the owners and ask whether the client/family gave informed consent to the placement decisions. This could be verified by meeting with the client/family to see if any questions concerning the OT recommendation of placements in a higher-

■ *Table 11.3.* **Analyzing Alternative Actions**

Action	Consequences	Ethical Principle
Quit in protest.	Owners hire another occupational therapist.	Fidelity to boss versus veracity
Meet with owners.	Owners tell occupational therapist to find another job.	Fidelity to boss versus veracity
	Owners agree to reconsider decision.	Nonmaleficence versus beneficence
	Owners assure occupational therapist that decision is in client's best interest.	Paternalism and cost-benefit versus autonomy and beneficence
	Owners assure occupational therapist it was a family decision.	Autonomy of client versus family
Meet with family.	Family has reasons for selecting current program.	Family versus individual power
	Family agrees with "least restrictive environment" approach.	Informed consent
Do nothing.	Occupational therapist is in violation of Code of Ethics, and possibly, of state and federal laws or regulations.	Duty; veracity to client; veracity to professional code, law, regulations

level setting remained. If the client and family believe that this setting is best for the client, then the therapist should respect their wishes. However, if the therapist believes that the family is acting on reasons other that the client's best interest and if this selection is detrimental to the client, further action is warranted. This action would involve reporting the proposed placement and decision-making process to the appropriate regulatory systems. This is an option that should be carefully examined prior to implementation.

If the family, upon receiving the information concerning the OT recommendation, decides that a higher-level placement is most appropriate, the owners should be informed of this decision. If the owners then engage in any inappropriate behavior, they should be reported by the family/therapist to the appropriate agency.

After this dilemma has been resolved, the therapist should meet again with the owners and seek assurances that the OT assessment will be used as part of the informed consent process of admission. If the owners are unable to make these assurances, it would appear that the therapist's and owners' methods and goals are in conflict. The therapist, realizing this, should seek an alternative employment opportunity. If the therapist has any knowledge of state regulations or laws being violated by the owners, the therapist is duty bound to report them.

Therapists rarely have to put their job on the line when faced with an ethical dilemma. If, when confronted with such a dilemma, therapists respond in a professional manner by using problem-solving and critical-thinking skills, most cases can be satisfactorily resolved.

However, if a situation exists where a client's rights or welfare are in jeopardy, the therapist cannot either ignore the situation or quit the job without confronting the situation. Either of these actions in certain circumstances could put the therapist in violation of the law (Hansen, Kamp, & Reitz, 1988).

To do a thorough analysis of an ethical dilemma and come to a comfortable resolution requires careful deliberation. The occupational therapist must take into consideration all of the factors that undergird the decision: personal and professional values, moral development, and the rights and duties of all the constituents. The occupational therapist needs to understand as much as possible about the context of the dilemma and then go about the process of finding a resolution (Hansen, 1990).

LEGAL ISSUES

The major emphasis in this chapter is the ethical issues involved in the evaluation and assessment process. I alluded to the importance of legal issues as well. There are some distinctions between what is ethical and what is legal. In many instances, the two are the same. That is because "(t)he law sets a baseline ethical standard for the community because the law, at least in a democratic republic, is a reflection of community values. (For example, everyone agrees that murder and rape are wrong ethically. It is such a common belief though, that we have statutes criminalizing such conduct)" (O'Neill, 1997, p. 3). However, there are situations when, although an action may be considered unethical, it might not be illegal. The converse is also true. For example, a practitioner who does not give credit to the creator of a noncopyrighted evaluation is behaving unethically but would not likely be charged in a court of law. Actions that might be illegal but ethical are complex in nature and not within the scope of this text. An example outside of the evaluation arena is the person who is a conscientious objector and refuses to enlist in the army. This person is acting ethically within his or her belief system; however, it is illegal to refuse to enlist.

An example of a conflict between ethical and legal action is when a report written to ensure that a client receives services. Some state or agency regulations require significant deficits before services can be instituted. However, the therapist may see a distinct need for intervention and, acting as an advocate for the client, may weight the deficit over any strengths observed to ensure that services are provided. This documentation of evaluation might be viewed as falsifying data for the "greater good" of the client. The action can be supported by ethical and moral beliefs, but it is technically illegal.

Two key points are: who may legally provide evaluations, and what is the amount that can be charged for these services? Providing evaluations that are within legal parameters is determined by several factors:

- the purpose of the assessment
- the state and federal laws that regulate practice
- the state, federal, and reimbursement regulations that determine payment
- the type of facility where the services are provided
- the formal and implicit contracts related to providing the assessment.

The occupational therapist should know and understand the regulations describing the scope of practice for occupational therapy and other professions in the state where he or she practices. If this state is one of the few states that have no regulation for occupational therapy practice, the regulations regarding payment (Medicare and Medicaid regulations and insurance contracts) will determine the appropriate credentials needed to legally bill for services. Another related issue is knowing and abiding by the stipulations of such contracts, regarding what services will be covered and how they should be billed. Only those assessments that are covered in the contract may be billed for payment.

Failure to know and abide by the laws that regulate occupational therapy practice may result in charges of malpractice. It could also lead to disciplinary action by the state regulatory board, state attorney general (Medicaid), or Federal Office of the Inspector General (Medicare). If there is evidence of criminal intent, the violator can be charged with fraud. Ignorance of the law is no excuse. We must be informed and alert to the legal context of practice that includes the process of evaluation (Hansen, 1990).

Summary

As with other aspects of the intervention process, evaluation and assessment require attention to the ethical and legal guidelines for good practice. This chapter contains a description of the development of personal and professional values and how they interrelate. *Core Values and Attitudes of Occupational Therapy Practice* (Kanny, 1993) and *Occupational Therapy Code of Ethics* (AOTA, 1994) are described and compared. The chapter provides a list of ethical considerations about evaluation from the perspective of the key players in the process. There is also a description of an analysis system to resolve ethical dilemmas, with a case example. Finally, there is a brief discussion of the differences and similarities between ethics and the law.

References

American Occupational Therapy Association. (1994). Occupational therapy code of ethics. *American Journal of Occupational Therapy, 48,* 1037–1038.

Aroskar, M.A. (1980). Anatomy of an ethical dilemma: The practice. *American Journal of Nursing, 4,* 661–663.

Gilligan, C. (1982). *In a different voice: Psychological theory and women's development.* Cambridge: Harvard University Press.

Hansen, R.A. (1990). Lesson 10: Ethical considerations. In C.B. Royeen (Ed.), *AOTA self study series. Assessing function.* Bethesda, MD: AOTA.

Hansen, R.A., Kamp, L., & Reitz, S. (1988). Two practitioners' analyses of occupational therapy practice dilemmas. *American Journal of Occupational Therapy, 42,* 312–319.

Hansen, R.A., & Kyler-Hutchison, P.L. (1989, April). Light at the end of the tunnel: Resolving dilemmas. Workshop presented at the American Occupational Therapy Association's Annual Conference, Baltimore, MD.

Hansen, R.A., Kyler-Hutchison, P.L., & Trompetter, L. (1994, October). Ethical issues and the health professions. *1994 Special Lecture Series.* College Misericordia, Occupational Therapy Program, Dallas, PA.

Kanny, E. (1993). Core values and attitudes of occupational therapy practice. *American Journal of Occupational Therapy, 47,* 1085–1086.

Kay, S.R. (1982). Kholberg's theory of moral development: Critical analysis of validation studies with the defining issues test. *International Journal of Psychology, 17,* 27–42.

Kohlberg, L. (1981). *Essays on moral development, Volume I, The philosophy of moral development.* San Francisco: Josey Bass.

Kurtines, W.M. & Gewirtz, J.L. (eds.). (1991). *Handbook of moral behavior and development* (Vols. 1–3). Hillsdale, NJ: Lawrence Erlbaum.

O'Neill, M. (1997, January). Reply to the Jehovah's Witness case. *Ethics in Formation, 7,* 3–5, 10–11.

Perry, W.G., Jr. (1970). *Forms of intellectual and ethical development in the college years: A scheme.* New York: Holt, Rinehart & Winston.

Rest, J.R. (1979). *Revised manual for the Defining Issues Test.* Minneapolis: University of Minneapolis.

Sparrow, S.S., Balla, D.A., & Cichetti, D.V. (1984). Vineland adaptive behavior scales. Circle Pines, MN: American Guidance Services.

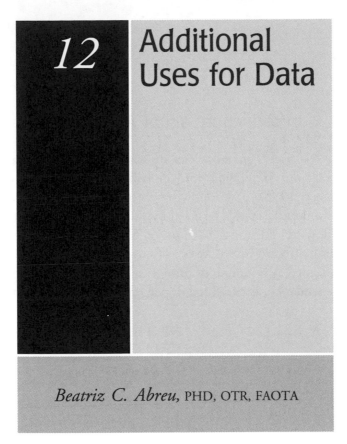

12 Additional Uses for Data

Beatriz C. Abreu, PHD, OTR, FAOTA

Overview

Data serve as a basis for decisions related to clinical, educational, and scientific investigations. Data assist practitioners in their thinking about the problems, questions, phenomena, or cases under investigation. Data are not a substitute for thinking. This chapter was motivated by the desire to open broader worlds of study, and to remind practitioners that all types of scientific inquiry, if adequately conducted, are rigorous and exciting. This chapter has been divided into nine sections:

1. Introduction: What are data?
2. How trustworthy and sound are data?
3. How can data be managed?
4. Data in scientific inquiry
5. Data in research
6. Data as central to documenting practice-based change
7. The rigor of qualitative data
8. The rigor of quantitative data
9. Outcome studies.

Every step of data usage is of great consequence to our clinical, academic, and scientific communities.

Introduction: What Are Data?

The term *data* has been defined as any information that serves as a basis for reasoning, discussion, calculation, and drawing conclusions (Norusis, 1986; Merriam-Webster, 1995). The following are examples of clinical data, both narrative and numerical, related to an individual named Edgar. Narrative data include the following: Edgar was born in 1975. He is right-handed, with both upper extremities affected by weakness. He was independent and happy until he had a head injury. A sampling of numerical data relates to Edgar's (patient 1) level of independence, as measured in percentages and shown in Table 12.1.

■ *Table 12.1.* Edgar's Level of Independence

Patient	ADL	Mobility	Meal Preparation	Money Management
1	100	80	90	75

Every occupational therapy student, practitioner, manager, educator, researcher, scholar, and philosopher uses such data.

Data management has been defined as the actions and operations needed for the systematic and coherent process of data collection, storage, and retrieval (Huberman & Miles, 1994). Systematic processes are needed to ensure that data are trustworthy and sound. These processes occur in three stages: before, during, and after data collection. A critical step before data collection is the careful formulation of the question to be answered and/or the identification of the phenomenon or case to be described, explained, or understood (Denzin & Lincoln, 1994; Norusis, 1986). This identification enables the user of data to decide exactly what pieces of information are necessary to solve the problem, answer the question, or understand the phenomenon or case under investigation. For example, a question we might ask about Edgar is, how much control does Edgar feel he has in the occupational therapy treatment? The pieces of information most relevant for answering this question must be narrative data.

Another consideration to make before data collection is the selection of data forms that may reduce collection errors. Occupational therapy practitioners obtain their information from standardized paper-pencil instruments, nonstandardized checklists, and other data forms developed in the field (Asher, 1996; Smith, 1992). The reader is referred to Chapters 5 and 6 for discussions of the process of gathering data from standardized and nonstandardized evaluations and assessments.

Data forms allow practitioners to systematically manage information for collection, storage, and retrieval. The occupational therapy literature is limited that provides guidelines for reviewing and preparing data forms and data bases from evaluations or assessments (Dijkers & Creighton, 1994; Renwick, 1991). Clear, simple, and well-organized data forms can minimize human, computer, or other measurement errors that can occur in the translation of information obtained from evaluative instruments when transcribing, coding, or keying information (Dijkers & Creighton, 1994; Smith, 1993; Weiss, 1990).

How Trustworthy and Sound Are Data?

Most therapists realize that the information gathered has to be "clean" in order for clinical, managerial, or research findings to be trustworthy. According to Dijkers & Creighton (1994), researchers in occupational therapy should follow data-cleaning strategies in order to prevent errors in analysis. In their discussion of data cleaning, these authors described errors related to instrumentation and human errors related to data processing. They named two categories of measurement errors: narrow sense and broad sense. Narrow sense errors describe those that relate to the *reliability* and *validity* of the data collection instruments, whereas broad sense errors refer to errors in data analysis, including the process of checking the accuracy of transcription, coding, and keying of data. These narrow and broad sense errors decrease the trustworthiness of research findings and the clinical decision-making process (refer to Figure 12.1). Therefore, correction of such errors can enhance the efficiency (cost/ time spent) and effectiveness (accuracy/validity of results) of both research and clinical outcomes (Dijkers & Creighton, 1994). Corrections for these errors require that a practitioner assess any tool's validity and reliability before recommending it for use.

As stated above, obtaining information about the reliability and validity of the instruments used is recommended to increase the trustworthiness of data. The reliability and validity of observations and methods are central issues for all scientific inquiry, irrespective of whether the approach is qualitative or quantitative (Kielhofner, 1982a). Reliability and validity for quantitative data are calculated as mathematical indices whereas the reliability and validity of qualitative data are determined largely in nonmathematical terms. The trustworthiness and soundness of the data will be examined later in this chapter.

Practitioners can obtain instrument validity and reliability indices by reviewing the literature or the protocol manual for that instrument. Two particular useful sources are the Twelfth Mental Measurement Yearbook (Conoley & Impara, 1995) and the *Occupational Therapy Assessment Tool: An Annotated Index* (2nd ed.) (Asher, 1996). In addition, practitioners and researchers can design standardized instruments and estimate their validity and reliability as part of their scientific inquiry. In the rehabilitation research literature, reliability indices are varied and are obtained using a variety of statistical methods (Portney & Watkins, 1993). Reliability indices such as interrater, test-retest, and internal consistency are estimated using statistical indexes such as Pearson Product Moment Correlation (P), Kappa (K), Percentage Agreement statistics, and Intraclass Correlation Coefficient (ICC).

Ottenbacker and Tomcheck (1993) noted that occupational therapists are likely to concerned themselves with *interrater reliability* frequently using Pearson Product Movement Correlations and Percentage Agreement indices. They note that the Pearson Product Movement Correlations and the Percentage Agreement indices are not adequate to measure interrater, intrarater, or test-retest agreement. Therefore, they advocate that the therapist should use the Intraclass Correlation Coefficient, or ICC, as a preferred index of reliability assessment. The ICC is considered a comprehensive reliability index that is able to provide assessment reliability measures in a variety of situations (Portney & Watkins, 1993). Further discussion of mathematical calculations and the methodological analysis of reliability is beyond the scope of this chapter.

How to Manage and Analyze Data

Huberman and Miles (1994) define *data management* as the procedure and operations needed for a systematic and coherent process of data collection, storage, and retrieval. They define *data analysis* as consisting of three sub-processes: data reduction, data display, and conclusion/verification. If we accept this definition for both quantitative and qualitative data, we can use the oversimplified diagram supplied in Figure 12.1.

DATA MANAGEMENT AND ANALYSIS

Computers are essential instruments for the effective and efficient management of information (Smith, 1993). The selection of the type of evaluation process, instrument, data form, or computer-assisted functions such as data collection, interpretation, and documentation, will reflect the level of clinical, research, and/or educational judgment of the data user. The computer's usefulness depends on the skill of the data user. Occupational therapists are expanding their use of technology for day-to-day operations in the clinic, classroom, and laboratory or field.

Data use is a complex process that requires systematic strategies that occur before, during, and after the collection, storage, retrieval, analysis, and interpretation of information. The type, amount, integrity, and appropriateness of data will represent a value system consisting of the data user's clinical, research, and educational judgments.

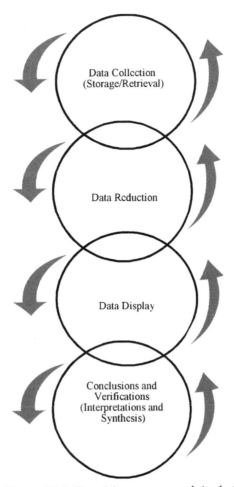

Figure 12.1. Data Management and Analysis

Many numerical data users employ computers in the application of data reduction and display, and use statistical procedures in order to integrate, synthesize, and make sense of data. A variety of computer software programs is available to assist therapists in the reduction, display, and analysis of data. Numerical data users employ programs such as Statistical Packages for Social Sciences (SPSS), Statistical Analysis System (SAS), and Crunch Interactive Statistical Package (CRUNCH). Computer software programs are also available to assist the therapist with the analysis of narrative or extended text data. Two popular programs are *The Ethnograph* (Siedel, 1988) and *Non-Numerical Unstructured Data Indexing, Searching, and Theory Building* (NUDIST) (Richards, 1987).

Although inductive reasoning has been associated primarily with qualitative research, because qualitative inquiry's type of analysis has been described as generative, constructive, and illuminative (Huberman & Miles, 1994), both qualitative and quantitative data can be analyzed using both inductive and

12.2. Differential Analysis for Numerical Versus Narrative Data

	Data Reduction
Narrative	Take notes on observations, field notes, tapes, site documents, objects, and people, using margin notes, longer reflective notes, and summary notes.
Numerical	Use mathematical calculations and computer software tools with commands to identify your data field, a command to specify how a data file should be read, and a command to indicate what you want to do with the data.
	Display of Data
Narrative	Use: 1) coding schemes; 2) data groups by color, by concepts, by metaphors, by numbers, by similarities, by differences, by reconstruction, or by deconstruction; 3) matrices according to time or effects.
Numerical	Use the average or arithmetic mean, median, mode, the variance, and standard deviations. Test hypotheses, evaluating differences between means.
	Verifications and Conclusions
Qualitative	Note relations between themes. Establish conceptual/theoretical coherence.
Quantitative	Note relations between variables. Establish conceptual/theoretical coherence and generalizations, interpret statistical tests, compare averages, rerun analysis, summarize results.

deductive reasoning. Many studies are based on a combination of inductive and deductive analysis. Data analysis in both quantitative and qualitative methodologies is sequential and interactive. In quantitative methodologies, the analysis of numerical data has a prescribed procedure. Qualitative methodologies, however, reflect an absence of investigator consensus in deciding the legitimate procedures for analysis and verification of narrative data. In an attempt to compare data analysis, Table 12.2 offers an oversimplified picture of selected methods for analyzing numerical data as well as data that are in extended text or narrative form.

WHAT ARE APPROPRIATE DATA?

The use of appropriate data is a critical component of direct care, education, and research. The appropriateness of systematic information is judged by the degree of suitability and usefulness of the data in answering questions and describing and explaining phenomena. In addition, data appropriateness is judged by the ethical considerations associated with the gathering of information. Each research methodology specifies guidelines for appraising the usefulness and suitability of data, in accordance with different assumptions. Data users who view qualitative methodologies favorably will declare that qualitative data are more appropriate than quantitative data for investigations in occupational therapy practice. The qualitative research orientation is viewed by some data users as more holistic and more in harmony than the quantitative research orientation with the goal of understanding the interpretations and meanings offered by individuals in their naturalistic sociohistorical environments (Carlson & Clark, 1991). Any judgment about the appropriate use of data will vary according to the attitude or opinion of the data user, which, in turn, is based on the question or problem under investigation. In the case of Edgar, the fact that he is right-handed is not so relevant as the fact that he was happy before his head injury.

Data in Scientific Inquiry

Occupational therapists use systematic methods of inquiry or investigation to generate new knowledge and to test the applications of knowledge in practice (Mosey, 1989, 1996; Zemke, 1989; Zemke & Clark, 1996a, 1996b). Theories are defined as plausible or scientifically acceptable principles offered to explain and predict phenomena (Merriam-Webster, 1995). For example, neurodevelopmental theory explains and predicts development. In this case, it is predicted that a child will be able to stand and walk after having achieved good head and trunk control. Empirical data constitutes information acquired by observation or practical experience (Merriam-Webster, 1995). For example, it is observed that a child may be able to stand and walk even in the presence of poor head and trunk control. Data users are capable of verifying or disproving empirical data by observation or experimentation.

All scientific inquiry includes logical reasoning, speculation, and interpretation. There are two types of scientific inquiry: 1) basic, which is concerned with the development or refinement of theories; and 2) applied, which relates to frames of references and guidelines for practice. Scientific inquiry may reflect the political bias of the researcher who is investigating and the community that accepts and promotes the findings (Clark et al., 1993; Mosey, 1993). For example, a graduate student from the University of Southern California may be positively biased towards research associated with the development of theory in occupational science, while a graduate student from New York University may be more accepting of applied research that is concerned with the development and testing of frames of reference.

All research studies reflect the beliefs, assumptions, and purposes of the researcher. The adapted diagram in Figure 12.2 illustrates parallels between qualitative and quantitative research methods.

DATA IN RESEARCH

Qualitative research represents a heterogenous approach that includes a variety of methodologies, such as phenomenological, life history, ethnographic, historical, and semiotic (Carlson & Clark, 1991; Krefting, 1991). Some occupational therapy researchers believe that qualitative methodologies can best enhance our knowledge of occupation and occupational therapy practice (Carlson & Clark, 1991; Kielhofner, 1982a, 1982b). Qualitative methodologies allow an

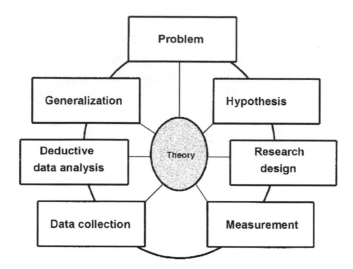

7 Steps for Quantitative Research

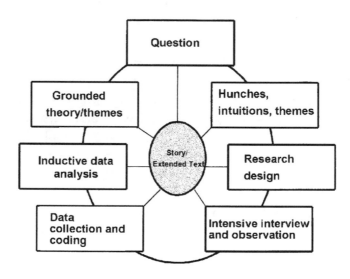

7 Steps for Qualitative Research

Figure 12.2. Parallels Between Qualitative and Quantitative Research Methods

Redrawn by permission from: Nachmias, D. and Nachmias, C. (1983) *Research methods in the social sciences* (2nd ed.), p. 23. NY: St. Martins Press, Inc. Adapted by Abreu, B. (1987)

investigator to understand another way of life from the participant's viewpoint (Krefting & Krefting, 1991). These methodologies also enable the examination of the social interdependence among individuals and their families, communities, ethnic traditions, and national cultures (Frank, 1996; Kielhofner, 1982a, 1982b). Occupational therapists can carefully examine the individual patterns of occupational selection and orchestration beyond a client-centered perspective (Frank, 1996). Researchers using qualitative methodologies can study occupational habits, perseverance, engrossment, flow, and termination (Carlson, 1996). These approaches can lead an investigator to understand the client's rehabilitation from a perspective beyond the confines of a specific occupational therapy intervention.

In qualitative analysis, the researcher employs manual or computer text-editing techniques in order to organize, identify the essential features of, and identify the interrelationships among the features for interpretation and meaningfulness of the data. These text-editing techniques include a systematic procedure of transforming data into a final account. Alasuutari (1995) describes qualitative analysis in the following manner: "Qualitative analysis differs in a number of respects. In it, the data are often considered as a totality; they are thought to shed light on the structure of a singular logical whole" (p. 11). Alasuutari posits that qualitative analysis consists of two phases: the purification of observations and unriddling. *Purification* refers to systematically thematizing the data from as many angles as possible. *Unriddling* means transforming the data into an explanation of the phenomenon being studied. Some qualitative researchers believe that analysis through computer software facilitates their interpretations (Weitzman & Miles, 1995). Others believe that computer analysis offers breadth but not depth (Seidel, 1992).

Quantitative research, on the other hand, involves the enumeration of numerical data about the individuals, phenomena, or units being studied. In order to organize and make data meaningful for description, interpretation, and inferences at the elemental level, the data user employs statistics (Ottenbacher, 1992b). Minium (1978) describes statistics as a field within the discipline of mathematics. Statistics employs techniques consisting of manual or computer-generated operations that transform data into a final account. The goal of quantitative research is to reduce the data so that the researcher can understand the relationship among defined variables.

It is the responsibility of the researcher to assess and justify the methodological rigor and ethical appropriateness of the data used during any investigation (Gliner, 1994; Johnston, Ottenbacher, & Reichardt, 1995; Yeaton & Sechrest, 1981). Occupational therapy is part science and part art, generating questions whose answer requires both qualitative and quantitative data. Ottenbacher (1992b) argues that there is confusion and contradiction in occupational therapy research because, at times, researchers subordinate the research problem to the methodology. He suggests that the discussions in our field "should focus on which research questions are important to occupational therapy rather than on how the question should be answered" (p. 871). In addition, he posits that both qualitative and quantitative methodologies are essential.

Data as Central to Documenting Practice-Based Change

Research and practice are seen as inseparable components for occupational therapy (Ottenbacher, Barris, & Van Deusen, 1986). In practice settings, practitioners must make decisions based on the data available. Documentation of meaningful, functional outcomes can be achieved with a variety of data.

Some therapists use statistics to organize and interpret numerical information obtained from the evaluation and intervention process. Statistical analysis of data allows the therapist to generate findings that describe the relationships among various pieces of data. The therapist is then able to interpret these findings to identify relationships, compare variables, or make predictions (Fink, 1995). A variety of analytical methods can be employed with numerical data including logistic regression, analysis of variance, and analysis of covariance.

Other therapists use different analytical methods to organize and interpret nonnumerical data. Nonnumerical data are words and multivoiced text including the descriptions, interpretations, representations, desires, and politics of the text (Denzin, 1994). Data analysis involves induction, content analysis, semiotics, and hermeneutics.

The information concerning the hypothetical figure Edgar at the start of this chapter included both kinds of data. Numerical data include Edgar's level of independence. Nonnumerical data include the words used in describing, explaining, and synthesizing information about him through systematic and prolonged observation and interviews. It also could include photographs, diaries, diplomas, and personal objects.

A variety of research methods can indeed support or be used to document practice-based change in an individual's performance. Before reviewing outcome research, the next sections further describe selected criteria contributing to sound qualitative and quantitative data. Although not every therapist has the resources or desire to do research, every therapist does have the obligation to participate in institutional accreditation processes that support the systematic and objective way of acquiring, collecting, and analyzing data for program evaluation, client satisfaction, and outcome evaluation and follow-up. The demand for systematic collection, analysis, and display of data from institutions offering occupational therapy services is inescapable. Therefore, knowledge of data use, both quantitative and qualitative, is critical for practice in the 1990s.

The Rigor of Qualitative Data

The specific qualitative research designs outline data collection, analysis, and interpretation. Qualitative researchers are concerned with the trustworthiness and credibility of their findings. Kielhofner (1982a, 1982b) describes how qualitative data undergo a metamorphosis of form and content during data gathering and data interpretation. He stresses that researchers should ensure that the "transformation process is not skewed or disturbed by instability in the data gathering phase or by a discontinuing between theoretical concept and its empirical concept" (p. 72). There are numerous techniques for ensuring rigor in the collection of qualitative data.

The qualitative researchers ensure the collection of credible data by addressing concerns that may influence the data they collect. For example, time or funding limitations may restrict the data collected (Spencer et al., 1993). Another issue is raised when a researcher is studying his or her own culture. In this case, the researcher's personal or professional roles may conflict with what he or she is discovering (Denzin, 1994). However, enhancement of practice has been reported from these studies. Mattingly and Gillette (1991) described a 2-year ethnographic study of occupational therapists at one hospital in which therapists and researchers collaborated. They reported an increase in clinical reasoning and an awareness of clinical success that was associated with the therapist's capacity to articulate assumptions, values, theories, and hypotheses about clinical practice. In all qualitative studies, researchers use several techniques to verify the data they collect.

Triangulation is a form of surveying information, a process through which different bearings give the correct position on and enhance credibility of the data (Silverman, 1993). As in the making of a triangle, determining two points (two perspectives) can allow one to locate a third point (third perspective) and view the total shape (total perspective). Triangulation includes a series of complementary methods of testing, comparing, supporting, or refuting the credibility of the final account of the data (Fielding & Fielding, 1986). The common classification described in the literature consists of four types of triangulation: of data, of investigator, of methods, and of theory.

Triangulation of data refers to the consistency of data about one individual performing in different contexts, times, and places (Fielding & Fielding, 1986; Krefting, 1991). Triangulation of data seeks to overcome the context-boundness of the information. Remember that qualitative data are explored and discovered in context (Figure 12.1).

Triangulation of methods is a multimethod approach. Two methods of triangulation are a within-method and a between-method. The first uses one method and employs multiple strategies to view the reliability of data. The second uses different methods on either different or the same subjects. If the different methods used show agreement, then the data show consistency and therefore have more credibility. There is controversy about using different triangulation design methods, because using different designs requires preplanning, a design characteristic not in harmony with qualitative research (Gliner, 1994; Lincoln & Guba, 1985).

Triangulation of investigators is used to evaluate the consistency of data; in this method different individuals examine the same qualitative data from the same situation to corroborate their credibility (Fielding & Fielding, 1986; Krefting, 1991). Gliner (1994) describes the process required in considering outliers (that data that are not completely consistent) as another way of attempting to corroborate the credibility of data when the investigators do not agree with the final account. This process is called *negative case analysis* (Lincoln & Guba, 1985; Patton, 1990).

The fourth type of triangulation used to determine credibility in qualitative research is called *triangulation of theory* or testing diverse or competing theories (Gliner, 1994; Lincoln & Guba, 1985). This method is controversial, because using different theories requires that the data be independent from theory—a logic not used in qualitative research, in which data are embedded in a theoretical perspective (Lincoln & Guba, 1985). However, Patton (1990) suggests that this process adds support to the credibility of data.

Other techniques for establishing credibility advanced by Huberman and Miles (1994) are the following: a *reflexivity journal*, in which the researcher explains the qualitative data collection methods, records, and reports, and includes decisions, data collection operations, database summary, analytic strategies, and key data displays that support the main conclusions. Another is an *audit* or review of evaluation studies. Huberman and Miles (1994) credit this method to Halpern (1983) and to Schwandt & Halpern (1988) with six rigorous questions to be evaluated and reported.

- Are findings grounded in the data? (Is sampling appropriate? Are data weighted correctly?)
- Are inferences logical? (Are analytic strategies applied correctly? Are alternative explanations accounted for?)
- Is the category structure appropriate?
- Can inquiry decisions and methodological shifts be justified? (Were sampling decisions linked to working hypotheses?)
- What is the degree of research bias (premature closure, unexplored data in field notes, lack of search for negative cases, feelings of empathy)?
- What strategies were used for increasing credibility (second readers, feedback to informants, peer review, adequate time in the field)? (p. 439)

The Rigor of Quantitative Data

The characteristics of research designs used in quantitative models of research determine the quality of the data findings, just as they do in qualitative approaches. A few quantitative design characteristics to be examined in this section are random assignment, effect size beyond statistical significance, and practical significance.

RANDOM ASSIGNMENT: BEYOND PREDETERMINATION

Random assignment is the designation of a procedure for predetermining the assignment of conditions to individuals in such a way that the chances for assignment to a particular condition are the *same* for all individuals (Otten-bacher, 1991a). Random assignment is used when the study requires equality between groups or conditions based on probability (Campbell & Stanley, 1963). Probability in this context refers to the branch of mathematics concerned with the study of certainty that a specific event or outcome will occur. For example, one might ask what the probability is that two groups of individuals receiving occupational therapy would have similar characteristics.

Random assignment is considered the best way to establish causation (Campbell & Stantley, 1963). Causation is the evidence of a relationship between the occurrence of some variations of one variable (for example, occupational therapy) and the production of subsequent changes in another variable (for example, independence in daily occupations) (Crano & Brewer, 1986). Relative to causation, one might ask what the probability is that occupational therapy interventions caused increased independence, if there is a change.

In quantitative research, variables are the things that are measured and represent the concepts studied. For convenience, variables are often classified as independent and dependent. One purpose of using random assignment, then, is to establish high standards of methodological rigor that can support or refute the effectiveness of the interventions studied. When experimental and nonexperimental designs deal with the determination of causation, the occupational therapy intervention may be referred to as the *cause* (or *independent variable*) and the outcome as the *effect* (or *dependent variable*).

ANALYSIS OF RANDOM ASSIGNMENT IN THE OCCUPATIONAL THERAPY LITERATURE

Ottenbacher (1995c) observed that if the methodological standards are not used, the results of the investigations will be considered uninterpretable from a scientific point of view, due to research design flaws. His recent research articles (1991d, 1992a, 1995a, 1995b) explain how individuals can use methodological standards in a manner that increases flexibility and relevance, while preserving appropriate design, accurate analysis, and clear interpretation of data. In 1991a, Ottenbacher reported on his examination of 44 research articles using group designs that had been published in the occupational therapy literature. His findings suggested that statistical significance was more frequently associated with designs that did not use random assignment.

Ottenbacher believes that the judgment about superior research design characteristics should not be conceptualized as consisting only of the predetermined factors (such as random assignment). Instead, he postulates that the quality of research studies can also be examined by testing research design characteristics after the fact, that is, as postdetermined events (Ottenbacher, 1991a). In this view, random assignment is seen as a moderator variable—as a method, factor, or characteristic that correlates with the size of the effect obtained in the various studies. When Ottenbacher compared random assignment as a moderator variable, he found that the studies using random versus nonrandom assignment were not that different. In his view, the quality of a research study can be seen in terms of its contribution to aggregated research outcome.

Therapist who have refrained from engaging in research because ethical or clinical considerations precluded a random assignment of subjects to groups should be encouraged by Ottenbacher's perspective. Practitioners are aware that random assignments in occupational therapy studies are difficult, unfeasible, and at times unethical (treatment vs. no treatment). These findings argue not against randomization but for a more flexible research design that enables problem-focused research versus methodology-focused research (Ottenbacher, 1992b).

DETERMINING EFFECT-SIZE: BEYOND STATISTICAL SIGNIFICANCE

The size of effect is a research design characteristic that is critical because the outcomes of a statistical test are strongly related to sample size (Ottenbacher, 1992c). The outcomes of a statistical test are determined to be either significant or not significant. Statistical significance occurs when the null hypothesis is rejected. The null hypothesis, represented as H_o, means that there is no treatment effect to be derived from the numerical value (scores) of the clients from two groups being compared. If there is a difference (for example, the group receiving a specific occupational therapy intervention has better scores), there is a treatment effect, and the null hypothesis (that there is no difference) is rejected. Inaccurate interference occurs when clinical significance is equated with statistical significance (Ottenbacher, Johnson, & Hojem, 1988). A way to minimize this misinterpretation is to insist on describing the interpretation of the data before the null hypothesis is tested by obtaining a p value. In addition, using size effect measures can also minimize the misinterpretation (Carver, 1993).

The *effect size* refers to the measures used to express the strength and magnitude of the findings that support the rejection of the null hypothesis or the degree to which a phenomenon is present in a population (Ottenbacher, 1992c; Sechrest & Yeaton, 1982). The *effect size* can be computed by using *eta squared* (Ottenbacher, 1992c). *Eta squared* is a measure that represents values independent of sample size and level of significance. This measure can be computed statistically from tests such as *F, t,* and *chi-square*.

Why Is the Effect Size Valuable?

The eta squared calculations can help occupational therapy researchers to determine the practical significance of the interventions studied and reported.

The reader is referred to Ottenbacher's articles to review the formula and the computation of various measures of effect size. Accurate clinical documentation about a client's progress requires that the research questions and design continue to be examined from the perspective of practical significance rather than only as statistically significant. Statistical significance depends on values such as p<.05, which is quite unrelated to clinical effect; however, both measures of statistical significance and effect size are important (Ottenbacher & Barrett, 1989).

Ottenbacher (1992c) examined the measures of effect for 237 statistical tests from 59 early intervention studies identifying the characteristics of research designs that answer the question of how much difference a particular program produced. His analysis supports the need to determine the *degree* of difference among groups and the relative impact of different interventions. He explains how traditional tests of statistical significance provide an all-or-none type of information regarding the null hypothesis (that there are no statistically significant differences). Further, he notes that statistical significance has limited value in defining the size of intervention effects for various programs, outcome measures, and populations. Therapists should be encouraged to determine practical significance in their studies. This practical significance can be supported by using single-subject or ideographic designs, as well as group comparisons or nomothetic designs (Ottenbacher, 1990).

Outcome Studies

Foto (1996) describes outcome studies as a "systematic procedure that allows us to evaluate the appropriateness, effectiveness, and efficiency of services we deliver as well as the degree to which those services meet the needs of our patients" (p. 87). Outcome research has increased in the 1990s. This major research undertaking requires a huge data base, consistency in data collection, and cooperative efforts in comparative data analysis. She enumerates four outcome measures that specify the questions to be asked about the degree of a client's progress as a result of therapy:

1. effectiveness
2. efficiency
3. quality
4. value (Foto, 1996).

Effectiveness measures can answer the question of which assessments and treatments produced the greatest functional gains. Efficiency measures can answer the question of which assessments and treatment timelines will produce, increase, and maintain the best results. Quality measures can answer the question of which assessments and treatments correlate with functional gain

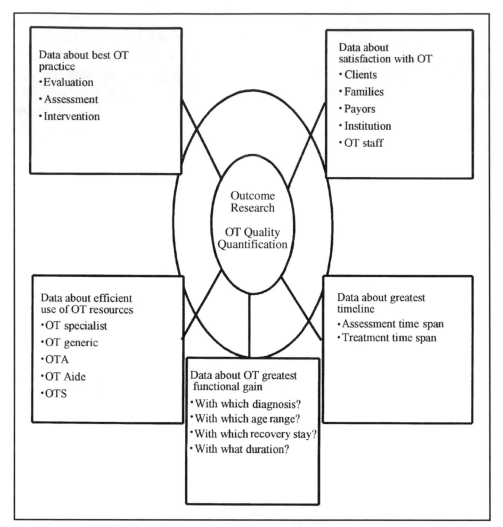

Figure 12.3. Outcome Research

and of what value or worth that gain is (see Figure 12.3). Value measures include the assessment of the client, the client's family, and the institution, regarding satisfaction with treatment and its contribution to prevention, cost containment, and service delivery (Ellenberg, 1996).

Many occupational therapists do not believe that we can accept or achieve the global outcome measure proposed by advocates of the socioethical model and by rigorous test and measurement agendas. Quality of life is not a stable and unified construct. For example, Velozo (1994) in his reflections about occupational therapy's selection of a single functional measure for outcome research wrote:

> The choice of a functional outcome measure for our profession is unlikely to be based on the measurement qualities of the instrument. Selection is more likely to be based on the industry standard (i.e.,

> the FIM). It is important, however, that the industry standard be sensitive enough to be the gold standard for occupational therapy. If we fall into the trap of choosing an instrument that is not a gold standard, we will have to live with the limitations of that instrument (p. 947).

He explains that if the outcome measures used in occupational therapy are not sensitive to the true functional level of clients upon their discharge from our services, we will not be able to capture the real effect of occupational therapy. The gold standard or ideal instrument needs to capture the real effect of our practice.

Relman (1988) believes that outcome studies have evolved from paradigm shifts in the American medical health care system that place a high priority on cost containment, assessment, and accountability. These priorities highlight the use of findings from outcome studies as the basis for health care reimbursement focusing on cost-effectiveness as well as quality-effectiveness (Van Leit, 1996). Data in outcome studies represent an attempt to quantify the quality of occupational therapy services and the efficacy of its science and art.

Peloquin (1996) reminds us that "management—skillful handling, direction, and control—is a function of care, but only a part of good care" (p. 456). This process requires that occupational therapists look carefully at the quantitative data (the numbers) obtained from outcome studies, as well as the qualitative data (the communications) that personalize programs and services. Five suggestions are:

1. Create occupational therapy programs that are considered good "package-deals" for the client, the payor system, as well as the occupational therapy department, because they attend to both outcome and process (Peloquin, 1996).
2. Study occupational therapy services systematically and publicize findings that include qualitative and quantitative data.
3. Educate occupational therapy staff in a variety of research methodologies.
4. Develop clinical pathways related to various diagnoses, follow them, reevaluate them, and assess their adequacy for meeting client's goals.
5. Educate client, family, and others about occupational therapy services to include evaluation, assessment, and treatment.

Ensuring a consumer's satisfaction with both process and outcome is a concern of all practitioners and administrators, and in particular of those professionals who practice case management. Case managers integrate the provision of care, coordinate efficient allocation of services, and ensure the consumer's satisfaction with process and outcomes (Malkmus & Johnson,

1992). Every therapist is indirectly an internal case manager for every client served.

Summary

Data use is a critical and inseparable component of direct care, education, and research. Careful selection of the problems, questions, or issues to answer and understand in occupational therapy practice is a complex process that requires knowledge, sophistication, and maturity. The acquisition and mastery of data for reasoning, discussion, calculation, and making conclusions about the art and science of practice is a developmental process. The process is colored by the experience, mentorships, and biases of occupational therapists. Recognition of the existence of methodological flaws, researcher biases, practice complexities, and imperfections with evaluation processes in occupational therapy leads us to cautious reflection.

It is not feasible or wise to advocate a singular method of data collection or system of analysis. On the contrary, this author believes in the multiplicity of voices that are present within the variety of qualitative and quantitative data methodologies. This multiplicity of voice and approaches requires discipline in its learning and further clarification in its teaching. Specific standards and criteria are necessary to help data users to judge the acceptability of data. Well-informed decisions and choices depend on data use. Our challenge is to provide clear, practical, and accessible literature on data use and on research methodology to readers in classrooms, clinics, and service organizations. In the world of research, the movement from novice to consumer and from consumer to expert requires work and nurturing. The statistical and nonstatistical bases for interpreting data in occupational therapy should relate to specific and relevant investigative issues and not to popularity, common use, or statistical or nonstatistical procedures promoted in the general research literature (Carver, 1993; Ottenbacher, 1990, 1991c, 1992a, 1992b, 1995c; Portney & Watkins, 1993). Data use in occupational therapy should advance the profession's practice, educational, and scientific missions.

ACKNOWLEDGMENT AND GRATITUDE

To Kenneth J. Ottenbacher, PhD, OTR, FAOTA for his numerous writings and help as a resource person offering guidelines for analysis and critique of data interpretation. To Suzanne M. Peloquin, PhD, OTR, for her editorial help and her inspirational voice in telling this story. And last but not least, to Dr. Brent Masel and the Moody Foundation for their support of this work.

References

Alasuutari, P. (1995). *Researching culture: Qualitative method and cultural studies.* London: Sage Publications.

Asher, I.E. (1996). *Occupational therapy assessment tools: An annotated index* (2nd ed.). Bethesda, MD: American Occupational Therapy Association.

Campbell, D.T., & Fiske, D.W. (1959). Convergent and discriminant validation by the multitrait-multimethod matrix. *Psychological Bulletin, 5b*, 81–105.

Campbell, D.T., & Stanley, J.C. (1963). *Experimental and quasi-experimental designs for research.* Chicago: Rand McNally.

Carlson, M. (1996). The self-perpetuation of occupations. In R. Zemke & F. Clark (Eds.), *Occupational science: The evolving discipline* (pp. 143–157). Philadelphia, PA: F.A. Davis.

Carlson, M.E., & Clark, F.A. (1991). The search for useful methodologies in occupational science. *American Journal of Occupational Therapy, 45*, 235–241.

Carver, N. (1993). The case against statistical significance testing. Revised. *Journal of Experimental Education, 61*, 287–292.

Clark, F., Zemke, R., Frank, G., Parham, D., Neville-Jan, A., Hedricks, C., Carson, M., Fazio, L., & Abreu, B. (1993). The issue is: Dangers inherent in the partition of occupational therapy and occupational science. *American Journal of Occupational Therapy, 47*, 184–186.

Conoley, J.C., & Impara, J.C. (Eds.). (1995). The twelfth mental measurement yearbook. Lincoln, NB: University of Nebraska.

Crano, W.D., & Brewer, M.B. (Eds.). (1986). *Principles and method of social research.* Boston, MA: Allyn and Bacon.

Crunch Interactive Statistical Package (CRUNCH) [Computer Software]. Oakland, CA: Crunch Software.

Denzin, N.K. (1994). The art and politics of interpretation. In N.K. Denzin & Y.S. Lincoln (Eds.), *Handbook of qualitative research.* Thousand Oaks, CA: Sage Publications.

Denzin, N.K., & Lincoln, Y.S. (1994). *Handbook of qualitative research.* Thousand Oaks, CA: Sage Publications.

Dijkers, M.P.J.M., & Creighton, C.L. (1994). Data cleaning in occupational therapy research. *Occupational Therapy Journal of Research, 14*, 145–156.

Ellenberg, D.B. (1996). Outcomes research: The history, debate, and implications for the field of occupational therapy. *American Journal of Occupational Therapy, 50*, 435–441.

Fielding, N.G., & Fielding, J.L. (1986). *Linking data* (Series 4). Newbury Park, CA: Sage Publications.

Fink, A. (1995). *How to analyze survey data.* Thousand Oaks, CA: Sage Publications.

Foto, M. (1996). Nationally speaking: Outcome studies: The what, why, how, and when. *American Journal of Occupational Therapy, 50*, 251–264.

Frank, G. (1996). Life histories in occupational therapy clinical practice. *American Journal of Occupational Therapy, 50*, 251–264.

Gliner, J.A. (1994). Reviewing qualitative research: Proposed criteria for fairness and rigor. *Occupational Therapy Journal of Research, 14*, 78–90.

Halpern, E.S. (1983). *Auditing naturalistic inquiries, some preliminary applications. Part 1: Development of the process. Part 2: Case study application.* Paper presented at the meeting of the American Educational Research Association.

Huberman, A.M., & Miles, M.B. (1994). Data management and analysis methods. In N.K. Denzin, & Y.S. Lincoln (Eds.), *Handbook of qualitative research* (pp. 428–444). Thousand Oaks, CA: Sage Publications.

Kielhofner, G. (1982a). Qualitative research: Part 1: Paradigmatic grounds and issues of reliability and validity. *Occupational Therapy Journal of Research, 2*, 67–79.

Kielhofner, G. (1982b). Qualitative research: Part 2: Methodological approaches and relevance to occupational therapy. *Occupational Therapy Journal of Research, 2,* 150–163.

Krefting, L. (1991). Rigor in qualitative research: The assessment of trustworthiness. *American Journal of Occupational Therapy, 45,* 214–222.

Krefting, L., & Krefting, D. (1991). Leisure activities after a stroke: An enthnographic approach. *American Journal of Occupational Therapy, 45,* 429–436.

Lincoln, Y.S., & Guba, E.G. (1985). *Naturalistic inquiry.* Beverly Hills, CA: Sage Publications.

Malkmus, D.D., & Johnson, P. (1992). Dedicated management of outcome, quality, and value: Internal case management. *Journal of Head Trauma Rehabilitation, 7 (4),* 57–67.

Mattingly, C., & Gillette, N. (1991). Anthropology, occupational therapy, and action research. *American Journal of Occupational Therapy, 45,* 972–978.

Merriam-Webster's Collegiate Dictionary (10th ed.). (1995). Springfield, MA: Merriam-Webster, Inc.

Minium, E.W. (Ed.). (1978). *Statistical reasoning in psychology and education* (2nd ed.). New York, NY: John Wiley & Sons.

Mosey, A.C. (1989). Editorial: The proper focus of scientific inquiry in occupational therapy: Frames of reference. *Occupational Therapy Journal of Research, 9 (4),* 195–201.

Mosey, A.C. (1992). The issue is: Partition of occupational science and occupational therapy. *American Journal of Occupational Therapy, 46,* 851–853.

Mosey, A.C. (1993). Partition of occupational science and occupational therapy: Sorting out some issues. *American Journal of Occupational Therapy, 47,* 751–754.

Mosey, A.C. (1996). *Applied scientific inquiry in the health professions: An epistemological orientation* (2nd ed.). Bethesda, MD: American Occupational Therapy Association.

Norusis, M.J. (1986). *The SPSS guide to data analysis.* Chicago, IL: SPSS, Inc.

Ottenbacher, K.J. (1986). An analysis of serial dependency in occupational therapy research. *Occupational Therapy Journal of Research, 6 (4),* 211–226.

Ottenbacher, K.J. (1990). Editorial: Occupational therapy curricula and practice: Skill based or knowledge based. *Occupational Therapy Journal of Research,* 7–11.

Ottenbacher, K.J. (1991a). Epistemology and experimentation of quality factors in research design. *American Journal of Occupational Therapy, 45,* 917–923.

Ottenbacher, K.J. (1991b). Interpretation of interaction factorial analysis of variance designs. *Statistics in Medicine, (10),* 1565–1571.

Ottenbacher, K.J. (1991c). Just do it. *Occupational Therapy Journal of Research, 11,* 131–1343.

Ottenbacher, K.J. (1991d). Statistical conclusion validity: An empirical analysis of multiplicity in mental retardation research. *American Journal of Mental Retardation, 95,* 421–427.

Ottenbacher, K.J. (1992a). Statistical conclusion validity and Type IV errors in rehabilitation research. *Archives of Physical Medicine and Rehabilitation, 73,* 121–125.

Ottenbacher, K.J. (1992b). Nationally speaking: Confusion in occupational therapy research: Does the end justify the method? *American Journal of Occupational Therapy, 46,* 871–874.

Ottenbacher, K.J. (1992c). Research methods. Practical significance in early intervention research: From affect to empirical effect. *Journal of Early Intervention, 16 (2),* 181–193.

Ottenbacher, K.J. (1995a). An examination of reliability in developmental research. *Development and Behavioral Pediatrics, 16 (3),* 177–182.

Ottenbacher, K.J. (1995b). The chi-square test: Its use in rehabilitation research. *Archives of Physical Medicine and Rehabilitation, 76,* 678–681.

Ottenbacher, K.J. (1995c). Why rehabilitation research does not work (as well as we think it should). *Archives of Physical Medicine and Rehabilitation, 76,* 123–129.

Ottenbacher, K.J., & Barrett, K.A. (1989). Measures of effect size in rehabilitation research. *American Journal of Physical Medicine and Rehabilitation, 68,* 52–58.

Ottenbacher, K.J., Barris, R., & VanDeusen, J. (1986). Some issues related to research utilization in occupational therapy. *American Journal of Occupational Therapy, 40,* 111–116.

Ottenbacher, K.J., Johnson, M.B., & Hojem, M. (1988). The significance of clinical change and clinical change of significance: Issues and methods. *American Journal of Occupational Therapy, 42,* 156–163.

Ottenbacher, K.J., & Stull, G.A. (1993). The analysis and interpretation of method comparison studies in rehabilitation research. *American Journal of Physical Medicine & Rehabilitation, 73,* 428–435.

Ottenbacher, K.J., & Tomchek, S.D. (1993). Reliability analysis in therapeutic research: Practice and procedures. *American Journal of Occupational Therapy, 47,* 10–16.

Patton, M.Q. (1990). *Qualitative evaluation and research methods* (2nd ed.). Newbury Park, CA: Sage Publications.

Peloquin, S.M. (1996). The issue is: Now that we have managed care, who shall inspire it? *American Journal of Occupational Therapy, 47,* 830–837.

Portney, L.G., & Watkins, M.P. (1993). Statistical measures of reliability. In L.G. Portney & M.P. Watkins (Eds.), *Foundations of clinical research applications to practice* (pp. 505–528). Norwalk, CT: Appleton & Lange.

Relman, A. (1988). Assessment and accountability: The third revolution in medical care. *New England Journal of Medicine, 319,* 1220–1222.

Renwick, R.M. (1991). A model for database design. *American Journal of Occupational Therapy, 45,* 827–832.

Richards, T.J. (1987). *User Manual for NUDIST: A text analysis program for the social sciences.* Melbourne, Australia: Replee, P/L.

SAS Institute (1979). *SAS user's guide.* Cary, NC: SAS Institute.

SPSS, Inc. (1983). *SPSS user's guide.* New York, NY: McGraw-Hill.

Schwandt, T.A., & Halpern, E.S. (1988). *Linking auditing and metaevaluation: Enhancing quality in applied research.* Newbury Park, CA: Sage.

Sechrest, L. & Yeaton, W.H. (1982). Magnitudes of experimental effects in social science research. *Evaluation Review, 6,* 579–599.

Seidel, J. (1988). *The Ethnograph* [Computer Software]. Littleton, CO: Qualis Research Associates.

Seidel, J.V. (1991). Method and madness in the application of computer technology to qualitative data analysis. In N.G. Fielding & R.M. Lee (Eds.), *Using computers in qualitative research* (pp. 107–116). Newbury Park, CA: Sage Publications.

Silverman, D. (1993). *Interpreting qualitative data: Methods for analyzing talk, text, and interaction.* London: Sage Publications.

Smith, R. (1992). Editorial: The science of occupational therapy assessment. *Occupational Therapy Journal of Research, 12 (1),* 3–15.

Smith, R.O. (1993). Computer-assisted functional assessment and documentation. *American Journal of Occupational Therapy, 47,* 988–992.

Spencer, J., Krefting, L., & Mattingly, C. (1993). Incorporation of enthnographic methods in occupational therapy assessment. *American Journal of Occupational Therapy, 47,* 303–309.

SYSTAT. (1990a). *Business MYSTAT: An instructional business version of SYSTAT for IBM-PC/compatibles*. Evaston, IL: Author.

SYSTAT. (1990b). *MYSTAT: An instructional version of SYSTAT for IBM-PC/compatibles*. Evanston, IL: Author.

Statistical Analysis System (SAS) [Computer Software]. Cary, NC: SAS Institute.

Statistical Packages for Social Scientists (SPSS) [Computer Software]. Chicago: SPSS.

Van Leit, B. (1996). Managed mental healthcare: Reflections in a time of turmoil. *American Journal of Occupational Therapy, 50*, 428–434.

Velozo, C.A. (1994). The issue is: Should occupational therapy choose a single functional outcome measure? *American Journal of Occupational Therapy, 48*, 946–947.

Weitzman, E.A., & Miles, M.B. (1995). *A software sourcebook: Computer programs for qualitative data analysis*. Thousand Oaks, CA: Sage Publications.

Yeaton, W.H., & Sechrest, L. (1981). Critical dimensions in the choice and maintenance of successful treatments: Strength, integrity, and effectiveness. *Journal of Consulting and Clinical Psychology, 49 (2)*, 156–167.

Zemke, R. (1989). The continua of scientific research designs. *American Journal of Occupational Therapy, 43*, 551–553.

Zemke, R., & Clark, F. (1996a). Preface. In R. Zemke & F. Clark (Eds.), *Occupational science: The evolving discipline* (pp. xii–xviii). Philadelphia, PA: F.A. Davis.

Zemke, R., & Clark, F. (1996b). Defining and classifying. In R. Zemke & F. Clark (Eds.), *Occupational science: The evolving discipline* (pp. 43–46). Philadelphia, PA: F.A. Davis.

Standards of Practice for Occupational Therapy

Preface

These standards are intended as recommended guidelines to assist occupational therapy practitioners in the provision of occupational therapy services. These standards serve as a minimum standard for occupational therapy practice and are applicable to all individual populations and the programs in which these individuals are served.

These standards apply to those registered occupational therapists and certified occupational therapy assistants who are in compliance with regulation where it exists. The term *occupational therapy practitioner* refers to the registered occupational therapist and to the certified occupational therapy assistant, both of whom are in compliance with regulation where it exists.

The minimum educational requirements for the registered occupational therapist are described in the current *Essentials and Guidelines of an Accredited Educational Program for the Occupational Therapist* (American Occupational Therapy Association [AOTA], 1991a). The minimum educational requirements for the certified occupational therapy assistant are described in the current *Essentials and Guidelines of an Accredited Educational Program for the Occupational Therapy Assistant* (AOTA, 1991b).

Standard I: Professional Standing

1. An occupational therapy practitioner shall maintain a current license, registration, or certification as required by law.
2. An occupational therapy practitioner shall practice and manage occupational therapy programs in accordance with applicable federal and state laws and regulations.
3. An occupational therapy practitioner shall be familiar with and abide by AOTA's (1994) *Occupational Therapy Code of Ethics* (*American Journal of Occupational Therapy, 48,* 1037–1038).
4. An occupational therapy practitioner shall maintain and update professional knowledge, skills, and abilities through appropriate continuing education or in-service training or higher education. The nature and minimum amount of continuing education must be consistent with state law and regulation.
5. A certified occupational therapy assistant must receive supervision from a registered occupational therapist as defined by official AOTA documents. The nature and amount of supervision must be provided in accordance with state law and regulation.
6. An occupational therapy practitioner shall provide direct and indirect services in accordance with AOTA's standards and policies. The nature and scope of occupational therapy services provided must be in accordance with state law and regulation.
7. An occupational therapy practitioner shall maintain current knowledge of the legislative, political, social, and cultural issues that affect the profession.

Standard II: Referral

1. A registered occupational therapist shall accept referrals in accordance with AOTA's *Statement of Occupational Therapy Referral* (AOTA, 1994) and in compliance with appropriate laws
2. A registered occupational therapist may accept referrals for assessment or assessment with intervention in performance areas, performance components, or performance contexts when individuals have or appear to have dysfunctions or potential for dysfunctions.
3. A registered occupational therapist, responding to requests for service, may accept cases within the parameters of the law.
4. A registered occupational therapist shall assume responsibility for determining the appropriateness of the scope, frequency, and duration of services within the parameters of the law.

5. A registered occupational therapist shall refer individuals to other appropriate resources when the therapist determines that the knowledge and expertise of other professionals is indicated.
6. An occupational therapy practitioner shall educate current and potential referral sources about the process of initiating occupational therapy referrals.

Standard III: Screening

1. A registered occupational therapist, in accordance with state and federal guidelines, shall conduct screening to determine whether intervention or further assessment is necessary and to identify dysfunctions in performance areas.
2. A registered occupational therapist shall screen independently or as a member of an interdisciplinary team. A certified occupational therapy assistant may contribute to the screening process under the supervision of a registered occupational therapist.
3. A registered occupational therapist shall select screening methods that are appropriate to the individual's age and developmental level; gender; education; cultural background; and socioeconomic, medical, and functional status. Screening methods may include, but are not limited to, interviews, structured observations, informal testing, and record reviews.
4. A registered occupational therapist shall communicate screening results and recommendations to appropriate individuals.

Standard IV: Assessment

1. A registered occupational therapist shall assess an individual's performance areas, performance components, and performance contexts. A registered occupational therapist conducts assessments individually or as part of a team of professionals, as appropriate to the practice settings and the purposes of the assessments. A certified occupational therapy assistant may contribute to the assessment process under the supervision of a registered occupational therapist.
2. An occupational therapy practitioner shall educate the individual, or the individual's family or legal guardian, as appropriate, about the purposes and procedures of the occupational therapy assessment.
3. A registered occupational therapist shall select assessments to determine the individual's functional abilities and problems as

related to performance areas, performance components, and performance contexts.

4. Occupational therapy assessment methods shall be appropriate to the individual's age and developmental level; gender; education; socioeconomic, cultural, and ethnic background; medical status; and functional abilities. The assessment methods may include some combination of skilled observation, interview, record review, or the use of standardized or criterion-referenced tests. A certified occupational therapy assistant may contribute to the assessment process under the supervision of a registered occupational therapist.

5. An occupational therapy practitioner shall follow accepted protocols when standardized tests are used. Standardized tests are tests whose scores are based on accompanying normative data that may reflect age ranges, gender, ethnic groups, geographic regions, and socioeconomic status. If standardized tests are not available or appropriate, the results shall be expressed in descriptive reports, and standardized scales shall not be used.

6. A registered occupational therapist shall analyze and summarize collected evaluation data to indicate the individual's current functional status.

7. A registered occupational therapist shall document assessment results in the individual's records, noting the specific evaluation methods and tools used.

8. A registered occupational therapist shall complete and document results of occupational therapy assessments within the timeframes established by practice settings, government agencies, accreditation programs, and third-party payers.

9. An occupational therapy practitioner shall communicate assessment results, within the boundaries of client confidentiality, to the appropriate persons.

10. A registered occupational therapist shall refer the individual to the appropriate services or request additional consultations if the results of the assessments indicate areas that require intervention by other professionals.

Standard V: Intervention Plan

1. A registered occupational therapist shall develop and document an intervention plan based on analysis of the occupational therapy assessment data and the individual's expected outcome after the intervention. A certified occupational therapy assistant may

contribute to the intervention plan under the supervision of a registered occupational therapist.

2. The occupational therapy intervention plan shall be stated in goals that are clear, measurable, behavioral, functional, and appropriate to the individual's needs, personal goals, and expected outcome after intervention.

3. The occupational therapy intervention plan shall reflect the philosophical base of occupational therapy (AOTA, 1979) and be consistent with its established principles and concepts of theory and practice. The intervention planning processes shall include
   a. Formulating a list of strengths and weaknesses.
   b. Estimating rehabilitation potential.
   c. Identifying measurable short-term and long-term goals.
   d. Collaborating with the individual, family members, other caregivers, professionals, and community resources.
   e. Selecting the media, methods, environment, and personnel needed to accomplish the intervention goals.
   f. Determining the frequency and duration of occupational therapy services.
   g. Identifying a plan for reevaluation.
   h. Discharge planning.

4. A registered occupational therapist shall prepare and document the intervention plan within the time frames and according to the standards established by the employing practice settings, government agencies, accreditation programs, and third-party payers. The certified occupational therapy assistant may contribute to the formation of the intervention plan under the supervision of the registered occupational therapist.

Standard VI: Intervention

1. An occupational therapy practitioner shall implement a program according to the developed intervention plan. The plan shall be appropriate to the individual's age and developmental level, gender, education, cultural and ethnic background, health status, functional ability, interests and personal goals, and service provision setting. The certified occupational therapy assistant shall implement the intervention under the supervision of a registered occupational therapist.

2. An occupational therapy practitioner shall implement the intervention plan through the use of specified purposeful activities or therapeutic methods to enhance occupational performance and achieve stated goals.

3. An occupational therapy practitioner shall be knowledgeable about relevant research in the practitioner's areas of practice. A registered occupational therapist shall interpret research findings as appropriate for application to the intervention process.

4. An occupational therapy practitioner shall educate the individual, the individual's family or legal guardian, non-certified occupational therapy personnel, and non-occupational therapy staff, as appropriate, in activities that support the established intervention plan. An occupational therapy practitioner shall communicate the risk and benefit of the intervention.

5. An occupational therapy practitioner shall maintain current information on community resources relevant to the practice area of the practitioner.

6. A registered occupational therapist shall periodically reassess and document the individual's levels of functioning and changes in levels of functioning in the performance areas, performance components, and performance contexts. A certified occupational therapy assistant may contribute to the reassessment process under the supervision of a registered occupational therapist.

7. A registered occupational therapist shall formulate and implement program modifications consistent with changes in the individual's response to the intervention. A certified occupational therapy assistant may contribute to program modifications under the supervision of a registered occupational therapist.

8. An occupational therapy practitioner shall document the occupational therapy services provided, including the frequency and duration of the services within the time frames and according to the standards established by the employing facility, government agencies, accreditation programs, and third-party payers.

Standard VII: Transition Services

1. The occupational therapy practitioner shall provide community-referenced services, as necessary, to identify occupational performance needs related to transition. Transition involves outcome-oriented actions which are coordinated to prepare or facilitate an individual for change, such as from one functional level to another, from one life stage to another, from one program to another, or from one environment to another.

2. The occupational therapy practitioner shall participate, when appropriate, in preparing a formal individualized transition plan based on the individual's needs and shall assist in the fulfillment

of life roles (e.g., independent or community living, self-care, care for others, work, play, and leisure) through activities in such a plan.

3. The occupational therapy practitioner shall facilitate the transition process in cooperation with the individual and the multidisciplinary team or other community support systems (including family members), when appropriate. The registered occupational therapist shall initiate referrals to appropriate community agencies to provide needed services (e.g., direct service, consultation, monitoring).

4. The occupational therapy practitioner shall determine the effectiveness of transition programs and the extent to which individuals have achieved desired transition outcomes (e.g., degree to which the individual is integrated and successful in community living and work environments). This is done in conjunction with the individual and other team members, where appropriate.

Standard VIII: Discontinuation

1. A registered occupational therapist shall discontinue service when the individual has achieved predetermined goals or has achieved maximum benefit from occupational therapy services.

2. A registered occupational therapist, with input from a certified occupational therapy assistant where applicable, shall prepare and implement a discharge plan that is consistent with occupational therapy goals, individual goals, interdisciplinary team goals, family goals, and expected outcomes. The discharge plan shall address appropriate community resources for referral for psychosocial, cultural, and socioeconomic barriers and limitations that may need modification.

3. A registered occupational therapist shall document the changes between the initial and current states of functional ability and deficit in performance areas, performance components, and performance contexts. A certified occupational therapy assistant may contribute to the process under the supervision of a registered occupational therapist.

4. An occupational therapy practitioner shall allow sufficient time for the coordination and effective implementation of the discharge plan.

5. A registered occupational therapist shall document recommendations for follow-up or reevaluation when applicable.

Standard IX: Continuous Quality Improvement

1. An occupational therapy practitioner shall monitor and document the continuous quality improvement of practice, which may include outcomes of services, using predetermined practice criteria reflecting professional consensus, recent developments in research, and specific employing facility standards.

2. An occupational therapy practitioner shall monitor all aspects of individual occupational therapy services for effectiveness and timeliness. If actual care does not meet the prescribed standard, it must be justified by peer review or other appropriate means within the practice setting. Occupational therapy services shall be discontinued when no longer necessary.

3. A registered occupational therapist shall systematically assess the review process of patient care to determine the success or appropriateness of interventions. Certified occupational therapy assistants may contribute to the process in collaboration with the registered occupational therapist.

Standard X: Management

1. A registered occupational therapist shall provide the management necessary for efficient organization and provision of occupational therapy services.

2. A certified occupational therapy assistant, under the supervision of a registered occupational therapist, may perform the following management functions:

   a. Education of members of other related professions and physicians about occupational therapy.

   b. Participation in (1) orientation, supervision, training, and evaluation of the performance of volunteers and other noncertified occupational therapy personnel, and (2) developing plans to remediate areas of skill deficit in the perfor-mance of job duties by volunteers and other noncertified occupational therapy personnel.

   c. Design and periodic review of all aspects of the occupational therapy program to determine its effectiveness, efficiency, and future directions.

   d. Systematic review of the quality of service provided, using criteria established by professional consensus and current research, as well as established standards for state regulation; accreditation; American Occupational Therapy Certification

Board (AOTCB) certification; and related laws, policies, guidelines, and regulations.

e. Incorporation of a fair and equitable system of admission, discharge, and charges for occupational therapy services.

f. Participation in cross-disciplinary activities to ensure that the total needs of the individual are met.

g. Provision of support (i.e., space, time, money as feasible) for clinical research or collaborative research when such projects have the approval of the appropriate governing bodies (e.g., institutional review board), and the results of which are deemed potentially beneficial to individuals of occupational therapy services now or in the future.

References

American Occupational Therapy Association. (1979). The philosophical base of occupational therapy. *American Journal of Occupational Therapy, 33,* 785.

American Occupational Therapy Association. (1991a). Essentials and guidelines of an accredited educational program for the occupational therapist. *American Journal of Occupational Therapy, 45,* 1077–1084.

American Occupational Therapy Association. (1991b). Essentials and guidelines of an accredited educational program for the occupational therapy assistant. *American Journal of Occupational Therapy, 45,* 1085–1092.

American Occupational Therapy Association (1994). Occupational therapy code of ethics. *American Journal of Occupational Therapy, 48,* 1037–1038.

American Occupational Therapy Association (1994). Statement of occupational therapy referral. *American Journal of Occupational Therapy, 48,* 1034.

Prepared by

Commission on Practice
Jim Hinojosa, PhD, OTR, FAOTA, Chairperson

Adopted by the Representative Assembly July 1994

Previously published and copyrighted by the American Occupational Therapy Association in the *American Journal of Occupational Therapy, 48,* 1039–1043.

Note: This document replaces the *1992 Standards of Practice for Occupational Therapy* (*American Journal of Occupational Therapy, 46,* 1082–1085) and the *1987 Standards of Practice for Occupational Therapy in Schools* (*American Journal of Occupational Therapy, 41,* 804–808), which were rescinded by the 1994 Representative Assembly.

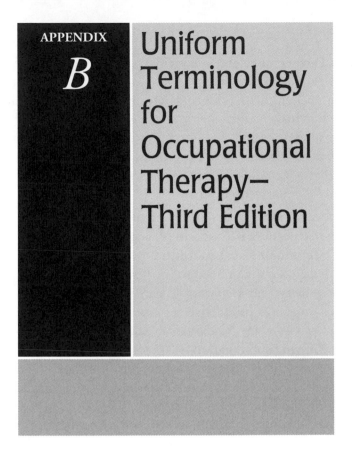

APPENDIX B

Uniform Terminology for Occupational Therapy— Third Edition

This is an official document of The American Occupational Therapy Association. This document is intended to provide a generic outline of the domain of concern of occupational therapy and is designed to create common terminology for the profession and to capture the essence of occupational therapy succinctly for others.

It is recognized that the phenomena that constitute the profession's domain of concern can be categorized, and labeled, in a number of different ways. This document is not meant to limit those in the field, formulating theories or frames of reference, who may wish to combine or refine particular constructs. It is also not meant to limit those who would like to conceptualize the profession's domain of concern in a different manner.

Introduction

The first edition of Uniform Terminology was approved and published in 1979 (AOTA, 1979). In 1989, *Uniform Terminology for Occupational Therapy—Second Edition* (AOTA, 1989) was approved and published. The second document presented an organized structure for understanding the areas of practice for the profession of occupational therapy. The document outlined two domains. **Performance areas** (activities of daily living [ADL], work and productive activities, and play or leisure) include activities that the occupational therapy practitioner emphasizes when determining functional abilities (*occupational therapy practitioner* refers to both registered occupational therapists and certified occupational therapy assistants). **Performance components** (sensorimotor, cognitive, psychosocial, and psychological aspects) are the elements of performance that occupational therapists assess and, when needed, in which they intervene for improved performance.

This third edition has been further expanded to reflect current practice and to incorporate contextual aspects of performance. **Performance areas**, **performance components**, and **performance contexts** are the parameters of occupational therapy's domain of concern. *Performance areas* are broad categories of human activity that are typically part of daily life. They are activities of daily living, work and productive activities, and play or leisure activities. *Performance components* are fundamental human abilities that—to varying degrees and in differing combinations—are required for successful engagement in performance areas. These components are sensorimotor, cognitive, psychosocial, and psychological. *Performance contexts* are situations or factors that influence an individual's engagement in desired and/or required performance areas. Performance contexts consist of *temporal* aspects (chronological age, developmental age, place in the life cycle, and health status) and *environmental* aspects (physical, social, and cultural considerations). There is an interactive relationship among performance areas, performance components, and performance contexts. Function in performance areas is the ultimate concern of occupational therapy, with performance components considered as they relate to participation in performance areas. Performance areas and performance components are always viewed within performance contexts. Performance contexts are taken into consideration when determining function and dysfunction relative to performance areas and performance components, and in planning intervention. For example, the occupational therapist does not evaluate strength (a performance component) in isolation. Strength is considered as it affects necessary or desired tasks (performance areas). If the individual is interested in homemaking, the occupational therapy practitioner would consider the interaction of strength with homemaking tasks. Strengthening could be addressed through kitchen activities, such as cooking and putting groceries away. In some cases, the practitioner would employ an adaptive approach and recommend that the family switch from heavy stoneware to lighter-weight dishes, or use lighter-weight pots on the stove to enable the individual to make dinner safely without becoming fatigued or compromising safety.

Occupational therapy assessment involves examining performance areas, performance components, and performance contexts. Intervention may be directed toward elements of performance areas (e.g., dressing, vocational exploration), performance components (e.g., endurance, problem solving), or the environmental aspects of performance contexts. In the latter case, the physical and/or social environment may be altered or augmented to improve and/or maintain function. After identifying the performance areas the individual wishes or needs to address, the occupational therapist assesses the features of the environments in which the tasks will be performed. If an individual's job requires cooking in a restaurant as opposed to leisure cooking at home, the occupational therapy practitioner faces several challenges to enable the individual's success in different environments. Therefore, the third critical aspect of performance is the performance context, the features of the environment that affect the person's ability to engage in functional activities.

This document categorizes specific activities in each of the performance areas (ADL, work and productive activities, play or leisure). This categorization is based on what is considered "typical," and is not meant to imply that a particular individual characterizes personal activities in the same manner as someone else. Occupational therapy practitioners embrace individual differences, and so would document the unique pattern of the individual being served, rather than forcing the "typical" pattern on him or her and family. For example, because of experience or culture, a particular individual might think of home management as an ADL task rather than "work and productive activities" (current listing). Socialization might be considered part of a play or leisure activity instead of its current listing as part of "activities of daily living," because of life experience or cultural heritage.

Examples of Use in Practice

Uniform Terminology—Third Edition defines occupational therapy's domain of concern, which includes performance areas, performance components, and performance contexts. While this document may be used by occupational therapy practitioners in a number of different areas (e.g., practice, documentation, charge systems, education, program development, marketing, research, disability classifications, and regulations), it focuses on the use of uniform terminology in practice. This document is not intended to define specific occupational therapy programs or specific occupational therapy interventions. Examples of how performance areas, performance components, and performance contexts translate into practice are provided below.

■ An individual who is injured on the job may have the potential to return to work and productive activities, which is a performance area. In order to achieve the outcome of returning to work and productive activities, the individual may need to address specific performance components, such as strength, endurance, soft tissue integrity, time management, and the physical features of performance contexts, like structures and objects in his or her environment. The occupational therapy practitioner, in collaboration with the individual and other members of the vocational team, uses planned interventions to achieve the desired outcome. These interventions may include activities such as an exercise program, body mechanics instruction, and job site modifications, all of which may be provided in a work-hardening program.

■ An elderly individual recovering from a cerebrovascular accident may wish to live in a community setting, which combines the performance areas of ADL with work and productive activities. In order to achieve the outcome of community living, the individual may need to address specific performance components, such as muscle tone, gross motor coordination, postural control, and self-management. It is also necessary to consider the sociocultural and physical features of performance contexts, such as support available from other persons, and adaptations of structures and objects within the environment. The occupational therapy practitioner, in cooperation with the team, utilizes planned interventions to achieve the desired outcome. Interventions may include neuromuscular facilitation, practice of object manipulation, and instruction in the use of adaptive equipment and home safety equipment. The practitioner and individual also pursue the selection and training of a personal assistant to ensure the completion of ADL tasks. These interventions may be provided in a comprehensive inpatient rehabilitation unit.

■ A child with learning disabilities is required to perform educational activities within a public school setting. Engaging in educational activities is considered the performance area of work and productive activities for this child. To achieve the educational outcome of efficient and effective completion of written classroom work, the child may need to address specific performance components. These include sensory processing, perceptual skills, postural control, motor skills, and the physical features of performance contexts, such as objects (e.g., desk, chair) in the environment. In cooperation with the team, occupational therapy interventions may include activities like adapting the student's seating in the classroom to improve postural control and stability, and practicing motor control and coordination. This program could be developed by an occupational therapist and supported by school district personnel.

■ The parents of an infant with cerebral palsy may ask to facilitate the child's involvement in the performance areas of activities of daily living and play. Subsequent to assessment, the therapist identifies specific performance components, such as sensory awareness and neuromuscular control. The practitioner also addresses the physical and cultural features of performance contexts. In collaboration with the parents, occupational therapy interventions may include activities such as seating and positioning for play, neuromuscular facilitation techniques to enable eating, facilitating parent skills in caring for and playing with their infant, and modifying the play space for accessibility. These interventions may be provided in a home-based occupational therapy program.

■ An adult with schizophrenia may need and want to live independently in the community, which represents the performance areas of activities of daily living, work and productive activities, and leisure activities. The specific performance categories may be medication routine, functional mobility, home management, vocational exploration, play or leisure performance, and social interaction. In order to achieve the outcome of living independently, the individual may need to address specific performance components, such as topographical orientation; memory; categorization; problem solving; interests; social conduct; time management; and sociocultural features of performance contexts, such as social factors (e.g., influence of family and friends) and roles. The occupational therapy practitioner, in cooperation with the team, utilizes planned interventions to achieve the desired outcome. Interventions may include activities such as training in the use of public transportation, instruction in budgeting skills, selection and participation in social activities, instruction in social conduct, and participation in community reintegration activities. These interventions may be provided in a community-based mental health program.

■ An individual with a history of substance abuse may need to reestablish family roles and responsibilities, which represent the performance areas of activities of daily living, work and productive activities, and leisure activities. In order to achieve the outcome of family participation, the individual may need to address the performance components of roles; values; social conduct; selfexpression; coping skills; self-control; and the sociocultural features of performance contexts, such as custom, behavior, rules, and rituals. The occupational therapy practitioner, in cooperation with the team, utilizes planned interventions to achieve the desired outcomes. Interventions may include roles and values exercises, instruction in stress management techniques, identification of family roles and activities, and support to develop family leisure routines. These interventions may be provided in an inpatient acute care unit.

Person–Activity–Environment Fit

Person–activity–environment fit refers to the match among the skills and abilities of the individual; the demands of the activity; and the characteristics of the physical, social, and cultural environments. It is the interaction among the performance areas, performance components, and performance contexts that is important and determines the success of the performance. When occupational therapy practitioners provide services, they attend to all of these aspects of performance and the interaction among them. They also attend to each individual's unique personal history. The personal history includes one's skills and abilities (performance components), the past performance of specific life tasks (performance areas), and experience within particular environments (performance contexts). In addition to personal history, anticipated life tasks and role demands influence performance.

When considering the person–activity–environment fit, variables such as novelty, importance, motivation, activity tolerance, and quality are salient. Situations range from those that are completely familiar to those that are novel and have never been experienced. Both the novelty and familiarity within a situation contribute to the overall task performance. In each situation, there is an optimal level of novelty that engages the individual sufficiently and provides enough information to perform the task. When too little novelty is present, the individual may miss cues and opportunities to perform. When too much novelty is present, the individual may become confused and distracted, inhibiting effective task performance.

Humans determine that some stimuli and situations are more meaningful than others. Individuals perform tasks they deem important. It is critical to identify what the individual wants or needs to do when planning interventions.

The level of motivation an individual demonstrates to perform a particular task is determined by both internal and external factors. An individual's biobehavioral state (e.g., amount of rest, arousal, tension) contributes to the potential to be responsive. The features of the social and physical environments (e.g., persons in the room, noise level) provide information that is either adequate or inadequate to produce a motivated state.

Activity tolerance is the individual's ability to sustain a purposeful activity over time. Individuals must not only select, initiate, and terminate activities, but they must also attend to a task for the needed length of time to complete the task and accomplish their goals.

The quality of performance is measured by standards generated by both the individual and others in the social and cultural environments in which the performance occurs. Quality is a continuum of expectations set within particular activities and contexts (see Figure 1).

Uniform Terminology for Occupational Therapy—
Third Edition

Occupational therapy is the use of purposeful activity or interventions to promote health and achieve functional outcomes. *Achieving functional outcomes* means to develop, improve, or restore the highest possible level of independence of any individual who is limited by a physical injury or illness, a dysfunctional condition, a cognitive impairment, a psychosocial dysfunction, a mental illness, a developmental or learning disability, or an adverse environmental condition. *Assessment* means the use of skilled observation or evaluation by the administra-

UNIFORM TERMINOLOGY FOR OCCUPATIONAL THERAPY
THIRD EDITION OUTLINE

I. Performance Areas

A. Activities of Daily Living
1. Grooming
2. Oral Hygiene
3. Bathing/Showering
4. Toilet Hygiene
5. Personal Device Care
6. Dressing
7. Feeding and Eating
8. Medication Routine
9. Health Maintenance
10. Socialization
11. Functional Communication
12. Functional Mobility
13. Community Mobility
14. Emergency Response
15. Sexual Expression
B. Work and Productive Activities
1. Home Management
a. Clothing Care
b. Cleaning
c. Meal Preparation/Cleanup
d. Shopping
e. Money Management
f. Household Maintenance
g. Safety Procedures
2. Care of Others
3. Educational Activities
4. Vocational Activities
a. Vocational Exploration
b. Job Acquisition
c. Work or Job Performance
d. Retirement Planning
e. Volunteer Participation
C. Play or Leisure Activities
1. Play/Leisure Exploration
2. Play/Leisure Performance

II. Performance Components

A. Sensorimotor Component
1. Sensory
a. Sensory Awareness
b. Sensory Processing
(1) Tactile
(2) Proprioceptive
(3) Vestibular
(4) Visual
(5) Auditory
(6) Gustatory
(7) Olfactory
c. Perceptual Processing
(1) Stereognosis
(2) Kinesthesia
(3) Pain Response
(4) Body Scheme
(5) Right-Left Discrimination
(6) Form Constancy
(7) Position in Space
(8) Visual-Closure
(9) Figure Ground
(10) Depth Perception
(11) Spatial Relations
(12) Topographical Orientation
2. Neuromusculoskeletal
a. Reflex
b. Range of Motion
c. Muscle Tone
d. Strength
e. Endurance
f. Postural Control
g. Postural Alignment
h. Soft Tissue Integrity
3. Motor
a. Gross Coordination
b. Crossing the Midline
c. Laterality
d. Bilateral Integration
e. Motor Control
f. Praxis
g. Fine Coordination/Dexterity
h. Visual-Motor Integration
i. Oral-Motor Control
B. Cognitive Integration and Cognitive Components
1. Level of Arousal
2. Orientation
3. Recognition
4. Attention Span
5. Initiation of Activity
6. Termination of Activity
7. Memory
8. Sequencing
9. Categorization
10. Concept Formation
11. Spatial Operations
12. Problem Solving 13. Learning
14. Generalization
C. Psychosocial Skills and Psychological Components
1. Psychological
a. Values
b. Interests
c. Self-Concept
2. Social
a. Role Performance
b. Social Conduct
c. Interpersonal Skills
d. Self-Expression
3. Self-Management
a. Coping Skills
b. Time Management
c. Self-Control

III. Performance Contexts

A. Temporal Aspects
1. Chronological
2. Developmental
3. Life Cycle
4. Disability Status
B. Environmental Aspects
1. Physical
2. Social
3. Cultural

Figure 1.

tion and interpretation of standardized or nonstandardized tests and measurements to identify areas for occupational therapy services.

Occupational therapy services include, but are not limited to

1. the assessment, treatment, and education of or consultation with the individual, family, or other persons; or
2. interventions directed toward developing, improving, or restoring daily living skills, work readiness or work performance, play skills or leisure capacities, or enhancing educational performance skills;
3. providing for the development, improvement, or restoration of sensorimotor, oral-motor, perceptual or neuromuscular functioning; or emotional, motivational, cognitive, or psychosocial components of performance.

These services may require assessment of the need for and use of interventions such as the design, development, adaptation, application, or training in the use of assistive technology devices; the design, fabrication, or application of rehabilitative technology such as selected orthotic devices; training in the use of assistive technology, orthotic or prosthetic devices; the application of physical agent modalities as an adjunct to or in preparation for purposeful activity; the use of ergonomic principles; the adaptation of environments and processes to enhance functional performance; or the promotion of health and wellness (AOTA, 1993, p. 1117).

I. Performance Areas

Throughout this document, activities have been described as if individuals performed the tasks themselves. Occupational therapy also recognizes that individuals arrange for tasks to be done through others. The profession views independence as the ability to self-determine activity performance, regardless of who actually performs the activity.

A. *Activities of Daily Living*—Self-maintenance tasks.
1. *Grooming*—Obtaining and using supplies; removing body hair (use of razors, tweezers, lotions, etc.); applying and removing cosmetics; washing, drying, combing, styling, and brushing hair; caring for nails (hands and feet), caring for skin, ears, and eyes; and applying deodorant.
2. *Oral Hygiene*—Obtaining and using supplies; cleaning mouth; brushing and flossing teeth; or removing, cleaning, and reinserting dental orthotics and prosthetics.
3. *Bathing/Showering*—Obtaining and using supplies; soap-

ing, rinsing, and drying body parts; maintaining bathing position; and transferring to and from bathing positions.

4. *Toilet Hygiene*—Obtaining and using supplies; clothing management; maintaining toileting position; transferring to and from toileting position; cleaning body; and caring for menstrual and continence needs (including catheters, colostomies, and suppository management).

5. *Personal Device Care*—Cleaning and maintaining personal care items, such as hearing aids, contact lenses, glasses, orthotics, prosthetics, adaptive equipment, and contraceptive and sexual devices.

6. *Dressing*—Selecting clothing and accessories appropriate to time of day, weather, and occasion; obtaining clothing from storage area; dressing and undressing in a sequential fashion; fastening and adjusting clothing and shoes; and applying and removing personal devices, prostheses, or orthoses.

7. *Feeding and Eating*—Setting up food; selecting and using appropriate utensils and tableware; bringing food or drink to mouth; cleaning face, hands, and clothing; sucking, masticating, coughing, and swallowing; and management of alternative methods of nourishment.

8. *Medication Routine*—Obtaining medication, opening and closing containers, following prescribed schedules, taking correct quantities, reporting problems and adverse effects, and administering correct quantities by using prescribed methods.

9. *Health Maintenance*—Developing and maintaining routines for illness prevention and wellness promotion, such as physical fitness, nutrition, and decreasing health risk behaviors.

10. *Socialization*—Accessing opportunities and interacting with other people in appropriate contextual and cultural ways to meet emotional and physical needs.

11. *Functional Communication*—Using equipment or systems to send and receive information, such as writing equipment, telephones, typewriters, computers, communication boards, call lights, emergency systems, Braille writers, telecommunication devices for the deaf, and augmentative communication systems.

12. *Functional Mobility*—Moving from one position or place to another, such as in-bed mobility, wheelchair mobility, transfers (wheelchair, bed, car, tub, toilet, tub/shower, chair,

floor). Performing functional ambulation and transporting objects.

13. *Community Mobility*—Moving self in the community and using public or private transportation, such as driving, or accessing buses, taxi cabs, or other public transportation systems.

14. *Emergency Response*—Recognizing sudden, unexpected hazardous situations, and initiating action to reduce the threat to health and safety.

15. *Sexual Expression*—Engaging in desired sexual and intimate activities.

B. *Work and Productive Activities*—Purposeful activities for self-development, social contribution, and livelihood.

1. *Home Management*—Obtaining and maintaining personal and household possessions and environment.

   a. *Clothing Care*—Obtaining and using supplies; sorting, laundering (hand, machine, and dry clean); folding; ironing; storing; and mending.

   b. *Cleaning*—Obtaining and using supplies; picking up; putting away; vacuuming; sweeping and mopping floors; dusting; polishing; scrubbing; washing windows; cleaning mirrors; making beds; and removing trash and recyclables.

   c. *Meal Preparation and Cleanup*—Planning nutritious meals; preparing and serving food; opening and closing containers, cabinets and drawers; using kitchen utensils and appliances; cleaning up and storing food safely.

   d. *Shopping*—Preparing shopping lists (grocery and other); selecting and purchasing items; selecting method of payment; and completing money transactions.

   e. *Money Management*—Budgeting, paying bills, and using bank systems.

   f. *Household Maintenance*—Maintaining home, yard, garden, appliances, vehicles, and household items.

   g. *Safety Procedures*—Knowing and performing preventive and emergency procedures to maintain a safe environment and to prevent injuries.

2. *Care of Others*—Providing for children, spouse, parents, pets, or others, such as giving physical care, nurturing, communicating, and using age-appropriate activities.

3. *Educational Activities*—Participating in a learning environment through school, community, or work-sponsored activities, such as exploring educational interests, attending to

instruction, managing assignments, and contributing to group experiences.

4. *Vocational Activities*—Participating in work-related activities.

   a. *Vocational Exploration*—Determining aptitudes; developing interests and skills, and selecting appropriate vocational pursuits.

   b. *Job Acquisition*—Identifying and selecting work opportunities, and completing application and interview processes.

   c. *Work or Job Performance*—Performing job tasks in a timely and effective manner; incorporating necessary work behaviors.

   d. *Retirement Planning*—Determining aptitudes; developing interests and skills; and selecting appropriate avocational pursuits.

   e. *Volunteer Participation*—Performing unpaid activities for the benefit of selected individuals, groups, or causes.

C. *Play or Leisure Activities*—Intrinsically motivating activities for amusement, relaxation, spontaneous enjoyment, or self-expression.

   1. *Play or Leisure Exploration*—Identifying interests, skills, opportunities, and appropriate play or leisure activities.

   2. *Play or Leisure Performance*—Planning and participating in play or leisure activities. Maintaining a balance of play or leisure activities with work and productive activities, and activities of daily living. Obtaining, utilizing, and maintaining equipment and supplies.

II. Performance Components

A. *Sensorimotor Component*—The ability to receive input, process information, and produce output.

   1. *Sensory*

      a. *Sensory Awareness*—Receiving and differentiating sensory stimuli.

      b. *Sensory Processing*—Interpreting sensory stimuli:

         (1) *Tactile*—Interpreting light touch, pressure, temperature, pain, and vibration through skin contact/receptors.

         (2) *Proprioceptive*—Interpreting stimuli originating in muscles, joints, and other internal tissues that give

information about the position of one body part in relation to another.

(3) *Vestibular*—Interpreting stimuli from the inner ear receptors regarding head position and movement.

(4) *Visual*—Interpreting stimuli through the eyes, including peripheral vision and acuity, and awareness of color and pattern.

(5) *Auditory*—Interpreting and localizing sounds, and discriminating background sounds.

(6) *Gustatory*—Interpreting tastes.

(7) *Olfactory*—Interpreting odors.

c. *Perceptual Processing*—Organizing sensory input into meaningful patterns.

(1) *Stereognosis*—Identifying objects through proprioception, cognition, and the sense of touch.

(2) *Kinesthesia*—Identifying the excursion and direction of joint movement.

(3) *Pain Response*—Interpreting noxious stimuli.

(4) *Body Scheme*—Acquiring an internal awareness of the body and the relationship of body parts to each other.

(5) *Right–Left Discrimination*—Differentiating one side from the other

(6) *Form Constancy*—Recognizing forms and objects as the same in various environments, positions, and sizes.

(7) *Position in Space*—Determining the spatial relationship of figures and objects to self or other forms and objects.

(8) *Visual-Closure*—Identifying forms or objects from incomplete presentations.

(9) *Figure Ground*—Differentiating between foreground and background forms and objects.

(10) *Depth Perception*—Determining the relative distance between objects, figures, or landmarks and the observer, and changes in planes of surfaces.

(11) *Spatial Relations*—Determining the position of objects relative to each other.

(12) *Topographical Orientation*—Determining the location of objects and settings and the route to the location.

2. *Neuromusculoskeletal*

a. *Reflex*—Eliciting an involuntary muscle response by sensory input.

    b. *Range of Motion*—Moving body parts through an arc.

    c. *Muscle Tone*—Demonstrating a degree of tension or resistance in a muscle at rest and in response to stretch.

    d. *Strength*—Demonstrating a degree of muscle power when movement is resisted, as with objects or gravity.

    e. *Endurance*—Sustaining cardiac, pulmonary, and musculoskeletal exertion over time.

    f. *Postural Control*—Using righting and equilibrium adjustments to maintain balance during functional movements.

    g. *Postural Alignment*—Maintaining biomechanical integrity among body parts.

    h. *Soft Tissue Integrity*—Maintaining anatomical and physiological condition of interstitial tissue and skin.

3. *Motor*

    a. *Gross Coordination*—Using large muscle groups for controlled, goal-directed movements.

    b. *Crossing the Midline*—Moving limbs and eyes across the midsagittal plane of the body.

    c. *Laterality*—Using a preferred unilateral body part for activities requiring a high level of skill.

    d. *Bilateral Integration*—Coordinating both body sides during activity.

    e. *Motor Control*—Using the body in functional and versatile movement patterns.

    f. *Praxis*—Conceiving and planning a new motor act in response to an environmental demand.

    g. *Fine Coordination/Dexterity*—Using small muscle groups for controlled movements, particularly in object manipulation.

    h. *Visual-Motor Integration*—Coordinating the interaction of information from the eyes with body movement during activity.

    i. *Oral-Motor Control*—Coordinating oropharyngeal musculature for controlled movements.

B. *Cognitive Integration and Cognitive Components*—The ability to use higher brain functions.

1. *Level of Arousal*—Demonstrating alertness and responsiveness to environmental stimuli.

2. *Orientation*—Identifying person, place, time, and situation.

3. *Recognition*—Identifying familiar faces, objects, and other previously presented materials.

4. *Attention Span*—Focusing on a task over time.

5. *Initiation of Activity*—Starting a physical or mental activity.

6. *Termination of Activity*—Stopping an activity at an appropriate time.
7. *Memory*—Recalling information after brief or long periods of time.
8. *Sequencing*—Placing information, concepts, and actions in order.
9. *Categorization*—Identifying similarities of and differences among pieces of environmental information)
10. *Concept Formation*—Organizing a variety of information to form thoughts and ideas.
11. *Spatial Operations*—Mentally manipulating the position of objects in various relationships.
12. *Problem Solving*—Recognizing a problem, defining a problem, identifying alternative plans, selecting a plan, organizing steps in a plan, implementing a plan, and evaluating the outcome.
13. *Learning*—Acquiring new concepts and behaviors.
14. *Generalization*—Applying previously learned concepts and behaviors to a variety of new situations.

C. *Psychosocial Skills and Psychological Components*—The ability to interact in society and to process emotions.
  1. *Psychological*
     a. *Values*—Identifying ideas or beliefs that are important to self and others.
     b. *Interests*—Identifying mental or physical activities that create pleasure and maintain attention.
     c. *Self-Concept*—Developing the value of the physical, emotional, and sexual self.
  2. *Social*
     a. *Role Performance*—Identifying, maintaining, and balancing functions one assumes oracquires in society (e.g., worker, student, parent, friend, religious participant).
     b. *Social Conduct*—Interacting by using manners, personal space, eye contact, gestures, active listening, and self-expression appropriate to one's environment.
     c. *Interpersonal Skills*—Using verbal and nonverbal communication to interact in a variety of settings.
     d. *Self-Expression*—Using a variety of styles and skills to express thoughts, feelings, and needs.
  3. *Self-Management*
     a. *Coping Skills*—Identifying and managing stress and related factors.
     b. *Time Management*—Planning and participating in a bal-

ance of self-care, work, leisure, and rest activities to promote satisfaction and health.

   c. *Self-Control*—Modifying one's own behavior in response to environmental needs, demands, constraints, personal aspirations, and feedback from others.

III. Performance Contexts

Assessment of function in performance areas is greatly influenced by the contexts in which the individual must perform. Occupational therapy practitioners consider performance contexts when determining feasibility and appropriateness of interventions. Occupational therapy practitioners may choose interventions based on an understanding of contexts, or may choose interventions directly aimed at altering the contexts to improve performance.

A. *Temporal Aspects*
1. *Chronological*—Individual's age.
2. *Developmental*—Stage or phase of maturation.
3. *Lifecycle*—Place in important life phases, such as career cycle, parenting cycle, or educational process.
4. *Disability status*—Place in continuum of disability, such as acuteness of injury, chronicity of disability, or terminal nature of illness.

B. *Environment*
1. *Physical*—Nonhuman aspects of contexts. Includes the accessibility to and performance within environments having natural terrain, plants, animals, buildings, furniture, objects, tools, or devices.
2. *Social*—Availability and expectations of significant individuals, such as spouse, friends, and caregivers. Also includes larger social groups which are influential in establishing norms, role expectations, and social routines.
3. *Cultural*—Customs, beliefs, activity patterns, behavior standards, and expectations accepted by the society of which the individual is a member. Includes political aspects, such as laws that affect access to resources and affirm personal rights. Also includes opportunities for education, employment, and economic support.

References

American Occupational Therapy Association. (1979). *Occupational therapy product output reporting system and uniform terminology for reporting occupational therapy services.* Bethesda, MD: Author.

American Occupational Therapy Association. (1989). Uniform terminology for occupational therapy—Second edition. *American Journal of Occupational Therapy, 43,* 808–815.

American Occupational Therapy Association. (1993). Association policies—Definition of occupational therapy practice for state regulation (Policy 5.3.1). *American Journal of Occupational Therapy, 47,* 1117–1121.

Prepared by

The Terminology Task Force
Winifred Dunn, PhD, OTR, FAOTA
Chairperson; Mary Foto, OTR, FAOTA
Jim Hinojosa, PhD, OTR, FAOTA
Barbara Schell, PhD, OTR/L, FAOTA
Linda Kohlman Thomson, MOT, OTR, FAOTA
Sarah D. Hertfelder, MEd, MOT, OTR/L, Staff Liaison
for
Commission on Practice
Jim Hinojosa, PhD, OTR, FAOTA, Chairperson

Adopted by the Representative Assembly July 1994

This document replaces the following documents, all of which were rescinded by the 1994 Representative Assembly: *Occupational Therapy Product Output Reporting System* (1979), *Uniform Terminology for Reporting Occupational Therapy Services—First Edition* (1979), "Uniform Occupational Therapy Evaluation Checklist" (1981, *American Journal of Occupational Therapy, 35,* 817–818), and "Uniform Terminology for Occupational Therapy—Second Edition" (1989, *American Journal of Occupational Therapy, 43,* 808–815).

Uniform Terminology– Third Edition: Application to Practice

Introduction

This document was developed to help occupational therapists apply *Uniform Terminology—Third Edition* to practice. The original grid format (Dunn, 1988) enabled occupational therapy practitioners to systematically identify deficit and strength areas of an individual and to select appropriate activities to address these areas in occupational therapy intervention (Dunn & McGourty, 1990). For the third edition, the profession is highlighting *contexts* as another critical aspect of performance. A second grid provides therapy practitioners with a mechanism to consider the contextual features of performance in activities of daily living (ADL), work and productive activity, and play or leisure. *Performance Areas* and *Performance Components* (see Figure A) focus on the individual. These features are imbedded in the *Performance Contexts* (see Figure B).

On the original grid (Dunn, 1988), the horizontal axis contains the Performance Areas of Activities of Daily Living, Work and Productive Activities, and Play or Leisure Activities (see Figure A). These Performance Areas are the functional outcomes that occupational therapy addresses. The vertical axis contains the Performance Components, including Sensorimotor components,

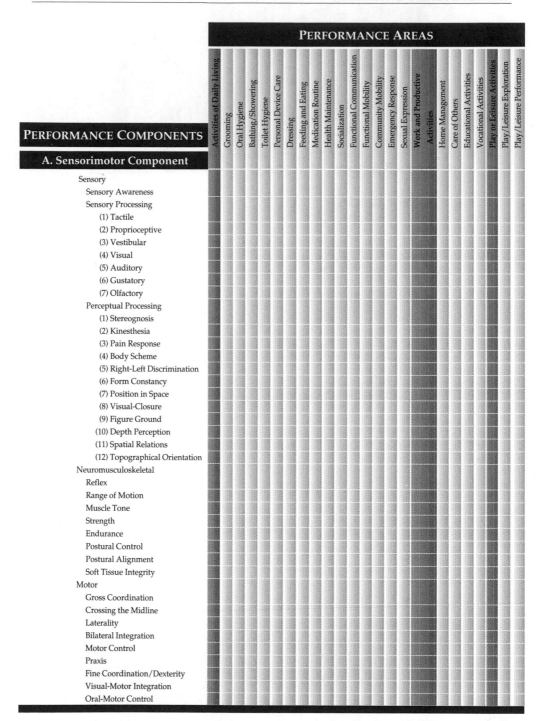

PERFORMANCE AREAS

Columns: Activities of Daily Living, Grooming, Oral Hygiene, Bathing/Showering, Toilet Hygiene, Personal Device Care, Dressing, Feeding and Eating, Medication Routine, Health Maintenance, Socialization, Functional Communication, Functional Mobility, Community Mobility, Emergency Response, Sexual Expression, Work and Productive Activities, Home Management, Care of Others, Educational Activities, Vocational Activities, Play or Leisure Activities, Play/Leisure Exploration, Play/Leisure Performance

PERFORMANCE COMPONENTS

A. Sensorimotor Component

Sensory
  Sensory Awareness
  Sensory Processing
    (1) Tactile
    (2) Proprioceptive
    (3) Vestibular
    (4) Visual
    (5) Auditory
    (6) Gustatory
    (7) Olfactory
  Perceptual Processing
    (1) Stereognosis
    (2) Kinesthesia
    (3) Pain Response
    (4) Body Scheme
    (5) Right-Left Discrimination
    (6) Form Constancy
    (7) Position in Space
    (8) Visual-Closure
    (9) Figure Ground
    (10) Depth Perception
    (11) Spatial Relations
    (12) Topographical Orientation
Neuromusculoskeletal
  Reflex
  Range of Motion
  Muscle Tone
  Strength
  Endurance
  Postural Control
  Postural Alignment
  Soft Tissue Integrity
Motor
  Gross Coordination
  Crossing the Midline
  Laterality
  Bilateral Integration
  Motor Control
  Praxis
  Fine Coordination/Dexterity
  Visual-Motor Integration
  Oral-Motor Control

Figure A. Uniform Terminology Grid (Performance Areas and Performance Components)

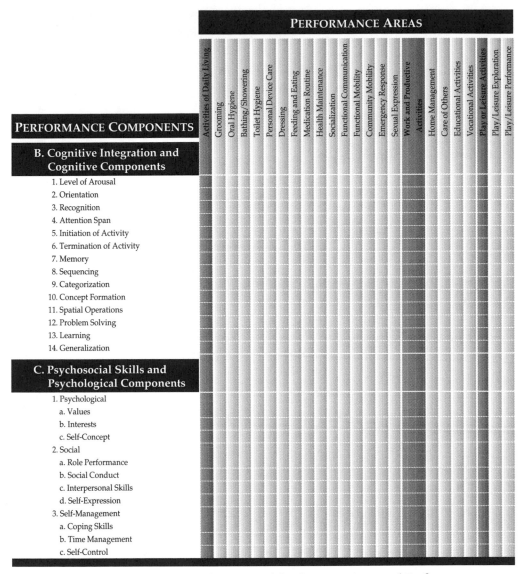

Figure A. Uniform Terminology Grid Continued (Performance Areas and Performance Components)

Cognitive Components, and Psychosocial Components. The Performance Components are the skills and abilities that an individual uses to engage in the Performance Areas. During an occupational therapy assessment, the occupational therapy practitioner determines an individual's abilities and limitations in the Performance Components and how they affect the individual's functional outcomes in the Performance Areas.

The first application document (Dunn & McGourty, 1989) described how to use the original *Uniform Terminology* grid with a variety of individuals. It is quite useful to introduce these concepts. However, the third edition of *Uniform Terminology* contains some changes in the Performance Areas and

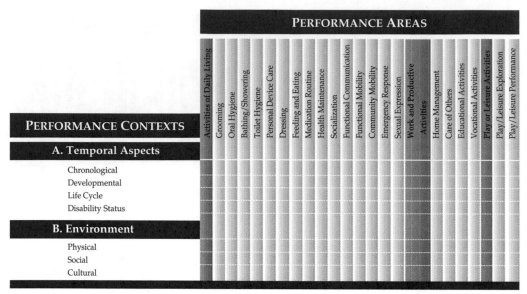

Figure B. Uniform Terminology Grid (Performance Areas and Performance Contexts)

Performance Components lists. Be sure to check for the terminology currently approved in the third edition before applying this information in current practice environments.

With the addition of Performance Contexts into *Uniform Terminology,* occupational therapy practitioners must consider how to interface what the individual wants to do (i.e., performance area) with the contextual features that may support or block performance. Figure B illustrates the interaction of Performance Areas and Performance Contexts as a model for therapists' planning.

The grid in Figure B can be used to analyze the contexts of performance for a particular individual. For example, when working with a toddler with a developmental disability who needs to learn to eat, the occupational therapy practitioner would consider all the Performance Contexts features as they might affect this toddler's ability to master eating. Unlike the grid in Figure A, in which the occupational therapy practitioner selects both Performance Areas (i.e., what the individual wants or needs to do) and the Performance Component (i.e., a person's strengths and needs), in this grid (Figure B) the occupational therapy practitioner only selects the Performance Area. After the Performance Area is identified through collaboration with the individual and significant others, the occupational therapy practitioner considers *all* Performance Contexts features as they might affect performance of the selected task.

Intervention Planning

Intervention planning occurs both within the general domain of concern of occupational therapy (i.e., uniform terminology) and by considering the profession's theoretical frames of reference that offer insights about how to approach the problem. In Figure A, the occupational therapy practitioner considers the Performance Areas that are of interest to the individual and the individual's strengths and concerns within the Performance Components. The intervention strategies would emerge from the cells on the grid that are placed at the intersection of the Performance Areas and the targeted Performance Components (strength and/or concern). For example, if a child needed to improve sensory processing and fine coordination for oral hygiene and grooming, an occupational therapy practitioner might select a sensory integrative frame of reference to create intervention strategies, such as adding textures to handles and teaching the child sand and bean digging games. Dunn and McGourty (1989) discuss this in more detail.

When using Figure B, the occupational therapy practitioner considers the Performance Contexts features in relation to the desired Performance Area. The occupational therapy practitioner would analyze the individual's temporal, physical, social, and cultural contexts to determine the relevance of particular interventions. For example, if the child mentioned above was a member of a family in which having messy hands from sand play was unacceptable, the occupational therapy practitioner would consider alternate strategies that are more compatible with their life-style. For example, perhaps the family would be more interested in developing puppet play. This would still provide the child with opportunities to experience the textures of various puppets and the hand movements required to manipulate the puppets in play context, without adding the messiness of sand. When occupational therapy practitioners consider contexts, interventions become more relevant and applicable to individual's lives.

Case Example 1

Sophie is a 75-year-old woman who was widowed 3 years ago, is recovering from a cerebrovascular accident (CVA), and has been transferred from an acute care unit to an inpatient medical rehabilitation unit. Prior to her admission, she was living in a small house in an isolated location and has no family living nearby. She was driving independently and frequently ran errands for her friends. She is adamant in her goal to return to her home after discharge. All of her friends are quite elderly and are not able to provide many resources for support.

Sophie and the team collaborated to identify her goals. Sophie decided that she wanted to be able to meet her daily needs with little or no assistance. Almost all of the Performance Areas are critical in order to achieve the outcome of community living in her own home. Being able to cook all of her meals, bathe independently, and have alternative transportation available is necessary. Because of their significant impact on the patient's function in the Performance Areas, some of the Performance Components that may need to be addressed are figure ground, muscle tone, postural control, fine coordination, memory, and self management.

In the selection of occupational therapy interventions, it is critical to analyze the elements of Performance Contexts for the individual. The physical and social elements of her home environment do not support returning home without modifications to her home and additional social supports being established. Railings must be added to the front steps, and provision of and instruction in the use of a tub seat and instruction in the use of specialized transportation may need to occur. If this same individual had been living in an apartment in a retirement community prior to her CVA, the contexts of performance would support a return home with fewer environmental modifications being needed. Being independent in cooking might not be necessary due to meals being provided, and the bathroom might already be accessible and safe. If the individual had friends and family available, the social support network might already be established to assist with shopping and transportation needs. The occupational therapy interventions would be different due to the contexts in which the individual will be performing. Interventions must be selected with the impact of the Performance Contexts as an essential element. ■

Case Example 2

Malcolm is a 9-year-old boy who has a learning disability that causes him to have a variety of problems in the school. His teachers complain that he is difficult to manage in the classroom. Some of the Performance Components that may need to be addressed are his self-control, such as interrupting, difficulty sitting during instruction, and difficulty with peer relations. Other children avoid him on the playground, because he does not follow rules, does not play fair, and tends to anger quickly when confronted. The Performance Component impairment with concept formation is reflected in his sloppy and disorganized classroom assignments.

The critical elements of the Performance Contexts are the temporal aspect of age appropriateness of his behavior and the social environmental aspect of his immature socialization. The significant cultural and temporal aspects of his family are that they place a high premium on athletic prowess.

The occupational therapy practitioner intervenes in several ways to address his behavior in the school environment. The occupational therapy practitioner focuses on structuring the classroom environment and facilitating consistent behavioral expectations for Malcolm by educational personnel. She also consults with the teachers to develop ways to structure activities that will support his ability to relate to other children in a positive way.

In contrast, another child with similar learning disabilities, but who is 12 years old and in the 7th grade might have different concerns. Elements of the Performance Contexts are the temporal aspect of the age appropriateness of his behavior and the social environmental context of school where bullying behavior is unacceptable and in which completing assignments is expected. In addressing the cultural Performance Contexts, the occupational therapy practitioner recognizes from meeting with parents that they have only average expectations for academic performance but value athletic accomplishments.

Since teachers at his school consider completion of home assignments to be part of average performance, the occupational therapy practitioner works with the child and parents on time management and reinforcement strategies to meet this expectation. After consultation with the coach, she works with the father to create activities to improve his athletic abilities. When occupational therapy practitioners consider family values as part of the contexts of performance, different intervention priorities may emerge. ■

Prepared by

The Terminology Task Force
Winifred Dunn, PhD, OTR, FAOTA, Chairperson
Mary Foto, OTR, FAOTA
Jim Hinojosa, PhD, OTR, FAOTA
Barbara A. Boyt Schell, PhD, OTR/L, FAOTA
Linda Kohlman Thomson, MOT, OTR, OT (C), FAOTA
Sarah D. Hertfelder, MEd, MOT, OTR/L, Staff Liaison
for
The Commission on Practice
Jim Hinojosa, PhD, OTR, FAOTA, Chairperson

This document replaces the 1989 document *Application of Uniform Terminology to Practice* that accompanied the *Uniform Terminology for Occupational Therapy—Second Edition* (*American Journal of Occupational Therapy, 43,* 808–815).

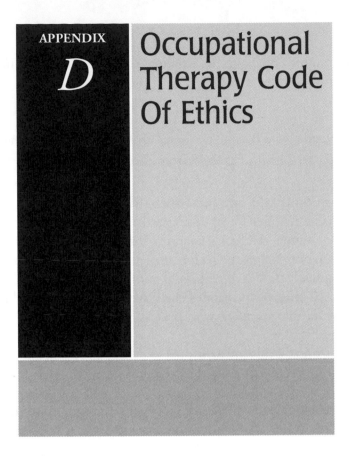

APPENDIX D

Occupational Therapy Code Of Ethics

The American Occupational Therapy Association's Code of Ethics is a public statement of the values and principles used in promoting and maintaining high standards of behavior in occupational therapy. The American Occupational Therapy Association and its members are committed to furthering people's ability to function within their total environment. To this end, occupational therapy personnel provide services for individuals in any stage of health and illness, to institutions, to other professionals and colleagues, to students, and to the general public.

The Occupational Therapy Code of Ethics is a set of principles that applies to occupational therapy personnel at all levels. The roles of practitioner (registered occupational therapist and certified occupational therapy assistant), educator, fieldwork educator, supervisor, administrator, consultant, fieldwork coordinator, faculty program director, researcher/scholar, entrepreneur, student, support staff, and occupational therapy aide are assumed.

Any action that is in violation of the spirit and purpose of this Code shall be considered unethical. To ensure compliance with the Code, enforcement procedures are established and maintained by the Commission on Standards and Ethics. Acceptance of membership in the American Occupational Therapy

Association commits members to adherence to the *Code of Ethics* and its enforcement procedures.

Principle 1. Occupational therapy personnel shall demonstrate a concern for the well-being of the recipients of their services. (beneficence)

A. Occupational therapy personnel shall provide services in an equitable manner for all individuals.

B. Occupational therapy personnel shall maintain relationships that do not exploit the recipient of services sexually, physically, emotionally, financially, socially or in any other manner. Occupational therapy personnel shall avoid those relationships or activities that interfere with professional judgment and objectivity.

C. Occupational therapy personnel shall take all reasonable precautions to avoid harm to the recipient of services or to his or her property.

D. Occupational therapy personnel shall strive to ensure that fees are fair, reasonable, and commensurate with the service performed and are set with due regard for the service recipient's ability to pay.

Principle 2. Occupational therapy personnel shall respect the rights of the recipients of their services. (e.g., autonomy, privacy, confidentiality)

A. Occupational therapy personnel shall collaborate with service recipients or their surrogate(s) in determining goals and priorities throughout the intervention process.

B. Occupational therapy personnel shall fully inform the service recipients of the nature, risks, and potential outcomes of any interventions.

C. Occupational therapy personnel shall obtain informed consent from subjects involved in research activities indicating they have been fully advised of the potential risks and outcomes.

D. Occupational therapy personnel shall respect the individual's right to refuse professional services or involvement in research or educational activities.

E. Occupational therapy personnel shall protect the confidential nature of information gained from educational, practice, research, and investigational activities.

Principle 3. Occupational therapy personnel shall achieve and continually maintain high standards of competence. (duties)

A. Occupational therapy practitioners shall hold the appropriate national and state credentials for providing services.

B. Occupational therapy personnel shall use procedures that conform to the Standards of Practice of the American Occupational Therapy Association.

C. Occupational therapy personnel shall take responsibility for maintaining competence by participating in professional development and educational activities.

D. Occupational therapy personnel shall perform their duties on the basis of accurate and current information.

E. Occupational therapy practitioners shall protect service recipients by ensuring that duties assumed by or assigned to other occupational therapy personnel are commensurate with their qualifications and experience.

F. Occupational therapy practitioners shall provide appropriate supervision to individuals for whom the practitioners have supervisory responsibility.

G. Occupational therapists shall refer recipients to other service providers or consult with other service providers when additional knowledge and expertise are required.

Principle 4. Occupational therapy personnel shall comply with laws and Association policies guiding the profession of occupational therapy. (justice)

A. Occupational therapy personnel shall understand and abide by applicable Association policies; local, state, and federal laws; and institutional rules.

B. Occupational therapy personnel shall inform employers, employees, and colleagues about those laws and Association policies that apply to the profession of occupational therapy.

C. Occupational therapy practitioners shall require those they supervise in occupational therapy related activities to adhere to the *Code of Ethics*.

D. Occupational therapy personnel shall accurately record and report all information related to professional activities.

Principle 5. Occupational therapy personnel shall provide accurate information about occupational therapy services. (veracity)

A. Occupational therapy personnel shall accurately represent their qualifications, education, experience, training, and competence.

B. Occupational therapy personnel shall disclose any affiliations that may pose a conflict of interest.

C. Occupational therapy personnel shall refrain from using or participating in the use of any form of communication that contains false, fraudulent, deceptive, or unfair statements or claims.

Principle 6. Occupational therapy personnel shall treat colleagues and other professionals with fairness, discretion, and integrity. (fidelity, veracity)

A. Occupational therapy personnel shall safeguard confidential information about colleagues and staff.

B. Occupational therapy personnel shall accurately represent the qualifications, views, contributions, and findings of colleagues.

C. Occupational therapy personnel shall report any breaches of the *Code of Ethics* to the appropriate authority.

Author

Commission on Standards and Ethics (SEC)
Ruth Hansen, PhD, OTR, FAOTA, Chairperson

Approved by the Representative Assembly April 1977
Revised 1979, 1988, 1994
Adopted by the Representative Assembly July 1994

Note: This document replaces the 1988 *Occupational Therapy Code of Ethics (American Journal of Occupational Therapy, 42,* 795–796), which was rescinded by the 1994 Representative Assembly.

Index

273

Fixed reference group, defined, 91
Forced choice, defined, 94
Form constancy, 256
Frame of reference, 5
    assessment tool, selection, 135–136
    as guide in interpretive process, 147–148
    phases of assessments, 138
    selection, 23–24
        assessment tool, 135–136
    theory, 24
    therapist's skills and perspective, 24
Freedom, defined, 199
Frequency distribution, defined, 91
Functional communication, 253
Functional mobility, 253
Functional Requirements in the Physical Environment, environmental assessment, 63

G

Generalization, 258
Generosity error, defined, 95
Goal attainment scaling, nonstandardized assessment, 122–123
Grade equivalent, defined, 91
Grooming, 252
Gross coordination, 257
Guttman scale, defined, 94

H

Halo effect, 83
    defined, 95
Health and Psychosocial Instruments (HaPI), standardized assessment, 102
Health maintenance, 253
Hierarchy of Competencies Relating to the Use of Standardized Instruments and Evaluation Techniques by Occupational Therapists, xiii
Home health, x
Home management, 254
Home Modification Workbook, environmental assessment, 63
Home Observation for Measurement of the Environment, environmental assessment, 63
Household maintenance, 254

I

Importance, Locus, and Range of Activities Checklist, environmental assessment, 63
Inclusion, ecology of human performance, 52–53
Independence

broad view, 53
    defined, 53
    ecology of human performance, 53–55
Independent Living Movement, ix
Individual error, defined, 86
Individual rights, 18
Inductive reasoning, assessment tool, 151
Infant-Toddler Environment Rating Scale, environmental assessment, 63
Information, dissemination, 4
Information processing, 149
Infra-team confidentiality, 14
Initiation of activity, 257
Interactive reasoning, 25–26, 149
Interests, 258
Internal consistency, defined, 88
Internet, standardized assessment, 102–103
Interobserver reliability, defined, 88
Interpersonal skills, 258
Interpersonal Support Evaluation List, environmental assessment, 64
Interrater reliability
    defined, 88
    nonstandardized assessment, 120
Intervention
    documentation, 168, 177
    Standards of Practice for Occupational Therapy, 239–240
Intervention planning
    philosophical assumptions, 147–148
    Standards of Practice for Occupational Therapy, 238–239
    Uniform Terminology for Occupational Therapy—Third Edition, 264–267
    case study, 265–267
Interview
    contextual evaluation, 71
    defined, 110
    nonstandardized assessment, 111–112
        in literature, 115
        strengths, 121
        weaknesses, 121
Intra-individual score differences, defined, 86
Intrarater reliability, defined, 88
Item analysis
    cross-validation, defined, 96
    item difficulty, defined, 96
    item discrimination, defined, 96
    Rasch analysis, defined, 96
    standardized assessment, 89–90, 95
Item bias, defined, 86
Item difficulty, item analysis, defined, 96
Item discrimination, item analysis, defined, 96